BEYOND THE MEDICAL MELTDOWN

ALSO BY DR. ROBERT ZIEVE

Healthy Medicine:
A Guide to the Emergence of Sensible, Comprehensive Care

BEYOND THE
MEDICAL MELTDOWN

Working Together for Sustainable Health Care

ROBERT J. ZIEVE, M.D.

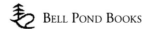 BELL POND BOOKS

BELL POND BOOKS
An imprint of Anthroposophic Press, Inc.
610 Main Street, Suite 1
Great Barrington, MA, 01230
www.steinerbooks.org

THE IMAGE ON THE FRONT COVER symbolizes the renewal of medicine. The commonly recognized symbol of medicine today, especially in the United States, is the caduceus, a rod with two entwined serpents and a pair of wings above. This commonly recognized symbol is related to the commercial side of modern medicine. It is this side of medicine that needs to be brought into balance with the deeper calling of medicine, which is healing. In this image, the caduceus resides within the tree, symbolizing strength and uprightness and connectedness with both the heavens and the earth. So it is that, to fulfill its purpose, medicine must help us to reestablish this sacred connectedness. Both tree and caduceus rest on the earth as a symbol of creating a more sustainable, effective, and affordable health care system that supports healing of the planet and its inhabitants.

FIRST EDITION

LIBRARY OF CONGRESS CATALOGING-IN-PUBLICATION DATA

Zieve, Robert J.
  Beyond the medical meltdown : working together for sustainable health care / Robert J. Zieve. — 1st ed.
    p. ; cm.
  Includes bibliographical references.
  ISBN-13: 978-0-88010-572-9
  ISBN-10: 0-88010-572-0
  1. Medical care. 2. Social medicine.   I. Title.
  [DNLM: 1. Healthcare Reform—trends—United States. 2. Delivery of Health Care—United States.   WA 540 AA1 Z67b 2006]
RA395.A3Z54 2006
362.1'0425—dc22
                                                        2006011202

CONTENTS

INTRODUCTION

BEYOND THE MEDICAL MELTDOWN: *Working Together for Sustainable Health Care* grew out of the many dialogues and interviews I have had since the publication of my previous book, *Healthy Medicine: A Guide to the Emergence of Sensible Comprehensive Care* (2005). The latter delineates for professionals and the general public how we can create health care that helps us all heal. It has universal and timeless application, but I recognized a need to address our current crisis more specifically.

Beyond the Medical Meltdown looks in more depth at where we are in the early twenty-first century and what we can and need to do to transform health care in the United States so that it is both effective and affordable. This book begins where *Healthy Medicine* left off. It provides the reader with a concise and accurate portrayal of our current health care dilemma, and then offers specific proposals for change that are common sense, practical, and imaginative.

Beyond the Medical Meltdown is for all who are experiencing the breakdown in health care: Medicaid recipients, government officials whose budgets are strained by Medicaid costs, businesses large and small that are under increasing financial strains from employer-based health insurance, retirees whose health care benefits have been cut by companies going out of business or whose co-pays have been increased by Medicare as it becomes heavily invested in pharmaceuticals, and everyone else who seeks health care.

In our daily news, we see evidence of a widespread social and cultural unraveling in such arenas as:

- Pharmaceutical and medical device company cover-ups
- Pension fund bailouts
- Bank and insurance company fraud
- Local community service collapses

And yet, as Margaret J. Wheatley, author of *Finding our Way*, has said in regard to reform of our social and financial systems, it is time to step away from that which does not work and begin to create that which works. This author agrees, and *Healthy Medicine* and *Beyond the Medical Meltdown* provide a model for stepping away from our current health care system and creating one that works instead.

I invite the reader to explore these pages with a mind and heart willing to see through the illusions of today, and willing to collaborate in creating health care that is both effective and affordable.

Lynne Twist, in her excellent book *The Soul of Money*, states that we are convinced of several beliefs that leave us feeling helpless. These include:

- There is not enough.
- More is better.
- Well, that's just the way it is.

Beyond the Medical Meltdown demonstrates that there is enough quality health care and enough money to pay for it, that more drugs and surgery is not necessarily better, and that the present health care quandary does not need to be the way it is. But to see this and to change health care will require enough people to wake up, think outside the box, and take action.

We are on a threshold. Health care as we have known it is dying. What we have come to see as "normal" medicine is not "healthy" medicine. We have, as Dr. John Abramson of Harvard phrases it, an "overdosed America" (see his book *Overdo$ed America*).

Health care today is a manipulated market, not a free market. It is neither effective nor affordable for most people in the United

States. In both the public sector and the private business world, it is a top-down, over-controlled system. This must change. *Beyond the Medical Meltdown* details how to create a bottom-up approach, which is necessary if health care is going to work for all of us.

So let's get started.

Chapter 1

MELTDOWN

HEALTH CARE TODAY is in a meltdown stage. Two trends are significantly squeezing putting pressure on an increasing number of people: rising health care costs and shrinking coverage. In discussing coverage, it is important to distinguish between coverage and good coverage. Insurance plans are covering ever fewer therapies and excluding almost all non-allopathic therapies. The result is worsening health care and worsening economics.

The former has produced an increase in chronic conditions. One example is the epidemic of diabetes, which is now affecting millions of Americans. Our current dependence on drugs and surgery will soon bankrupt our health care system if it continues on this present course, a course that is becoming more rigid as it is being controlled by fewer decision makers. How did we get to this point?

The 1990s

In the 1990s, two events occurred that accelerated the health care crisis and helped bring us to our current predicament. These events were: Medical expenses exceeded inflation, and managed care insurance companies limited patient treatment options.

1. MEDICAL EXPENSES EXCEEDED INFLATION.

This occurred because of increasing demand and because more expensive and often unnecessary technologies were introduced and became commonplace. If this continues, what awaits us is a future of worsening personal health and worsening economic health of cities and states. These expensive new technologies include:

- Cardiovascular techniques such as bypass surgeries, stents, heart valves, and other invasive procedures.
- Drugs such as statins and new generation cancer drugs. The former mislead the general public into thinking that lowering blood cholesterol translates into lower risk of coronary artery disease, which it doesn't. The latter are building up a record of financial greed, with the claim of prolonging a life for a year or so at a cost of more than $200,000, at great suffering from side effects, and often with unproven efficacy, when there are many effective cancer therapies known worldwide in the field of what the medical establishment often derisively terms "alternative" medicine.

Again, some of these technologies are needed some of the time. But in a system of fully comprehensive medicine (which I define as medicine that integrates all fields of medicine and healing into a unified, comprehensive whole), as described in *Healthy Medicine,* these approaches would be called on less and less. The reader must perceive how the regular medical system with its built-in legal and financial protections is artificially driving up health care costs, at the expense of local communities that are forced to close libraries in order to finance Medicaid, and at the expense of individuals who are forced into bankruptcy by medical costs.

2. Managed care insurance companies limited patient treatment options.

Allowable treatments options were, of course, only those of allopathic or conventional medicine. This limiting creates a fear and scarcity mentality. It is a mentality that is false, but exists because of the artificial financing and overdependence on conventional medicine.

These two developments in health care are clear examples of a wrong allocation of resources due to narrow-minded and greed-driven thinking and financial manipulation of the holy profession of medicine. Health care today is essentially a rationing by the "free market" composed of insurance companies, hospitals, medical supply companies, and pharmaceutical companies, in collusion with government. This rationing has been built into our legal structures and organized medicine.

In the 1990s, in no small part due to highly effective advertising, the consumer of health care wanted more choice, and that choice meant more expensive therapies and testing. Again, the weakness of America: More = Better. And in this country, choice means freedom. The ideal of freedom of choice clearly ran into conflict with the perception that managed care companies were the bad guys, limiting people's choices of health care. But the problem with this simplistic approach is the perception that everyone should have the freedom to choose his own health care, regardless of the expense, and have managed care or government pay for it. This approach lacks the element of personal responsibility for changing illness-generating lifestyle habits. The lessons here are:

- There is no freedom without responsibility.
- Responsibility extends to everyone: patients, health care practitioners, and corporations in health care. Each of these players is hiding and shuffling, in their own way.

The results of these 1990s trends were: Higher out of pocket costs for the health care people demand.

- Cost-shifting: the sicker pay more for health care, and more often than not, the sicker are poorer, on Medicaid, or uninsured.

After the Millennium

The ongoing perpetuation of governmental and private insurance funding of conventional medicine to the virtual exclusion of alternative/complementary medicine has led to three consequences:

1. A dramatic increase in many chronic debilitating diseases that drugs and surgery will never heal. More people will suffer unnecessarily.

2. A bankrupting of governmental capacities at all levels to provide effective health care services. This will be accelerated with the new Medicare drug-financing law that is taking effect soon, in accordance with which the government will underwrite billions of dollars being spent to provide pharmaceutical drugs to Medicare patients. This will ultimately lead to unnecessary increases in health care costs because of the virtually exclusive financing of pharmaceutical medicine and the exclusion of natural medicine. Because of the rising costs associated with allopathically financed treatment of chronic illness, this new law will further undermine effective government support of other necessary and vital services.

3. An increase in financial stress on individuals and families, as people stay in jobs that provide decreasing health care coverage, with higher deductibles, for services that do not help heal, and more often than not lead to further chronic illness.

Like many other institutions in America, medicine today lusts for profit for profit's sake. Although this may not be immediately apparent when you go to the doctor's office, it is the reality behind the scenes in the medical industrial complex that now dominates health care. That reality has brought health care to a state of near breakdown. The critical condition in which we now find ourselves is evident in a number of different areas of our economy: company retiree benefits, local government deficits, Medicare, and employer-based health care insurance.

Company Retiree Benefits

More and more companies are declaring they no longer have the funds to pay for the health care needs of retirees. These were funds that employees trusted would be there to help them afford medical care after retirement, when health care costs are usually more than in working years. Bethlehem Steel and United Airlines are among the companies that have stopped paying into their pension plans. This has forced the government to step in and assume responsibility for these corporate commitments to employees, at taxpayer expense, and most often at much less of a financial commitment to retiree's than was the original company commitment

Local Government Deficits

Government is the single biggest player and payer of health care. Yet today we find so much debt and so little money to meet human social needs like health care. Small and medium-sized communities throughout the United States are being forced to cut such essential and community-supportive projects as public libraries, arts education, parks, and other similar areas of public life that we have come to take for granted. This is occurring because of the tremendous financial strain that is now on local and regional governments due to the health care benefits they must fund. These benefits take a number of forms, but two major ones are pension funds for government retirees and Medicaid Medicare is a state and federal joint effort, whereas Medicare is a federal program.

Many states and cities throughout the United States are facing pension obligations that are already large and growing larger. The increasing financial strain of these obligations is forcing all levels of government to cut other basic services such as health care and education. This strain can only worsen as these pension obligations grow.

Medicaid and pension funding are individually putting a tremendous strain on healthy local economies. Together they are threatening to bankrupt these economies in the very near future. In some areas of the country, this is already happening.

The *New York Times* reported (December 26, 2005) that the recent transit strike in New York City brought to the surface commitments made decades ago by city and state governments to fund health care benefits for retirees, in addition to pension funds. New accounting rules that go into effect in 2006, which are finally going to provide a truer accounting of this issue, reveal that the cost to the city for retiree health care benefits will rise from less than one billion dollars to between five and ten billion dollars. According to the article, "The pay-as-you-go accounting method that New York now uses greatly understates the full obligation taxpayers have incurred because it does not include any benefits to be paid in the future. Most other state and local governments that offer significant health benefits to retirees use the same method and will also have to bring newer, larger numbers onto their books in the next two or three years."

If cities are forced to raise taxes and/or cut benefits to pay for these increased costs, how will the residents respond?

DULUTH, MINNESOTA: A MICROCOSM OF THE NATION

Duluth and many other cities are facing what is called an economic time bomb in the form of health care benefits for retirees. In an earlier time, these were promised for free as part of the social contract of that time. When this time bomb is combined with health insurance expenditures for current employees and their families and increasing Medicaid costs, the magnitude of the crisis starts to become obvious. Among the components of the economic time bomb that Duluth, which is representative of the situation throughout the United States, is facing are:

- Growth in health care expenses because of overdependence on pharmaceuticals and hospital-based interventions
- Worsening health of the general population, in comparison to two generations ago. This is due to many factors, including a

plethora of environmental toxins and a multitude of nutritional deficiencies from poor diets, that is, diets dependent on fast foods.

- Internal stress of many employees, due to factors such as financial stress, poor health, and workplace conditions.
- A health care economy that has permitted millions of dollars to be hidden by accounting methods. These unrecorded liabilities are coming home to roost.
- Stock-market portfolios in which cities have invested pension funds losing their value.
- A greedy health care industry that is much more focused on profits and returns to investors than on healing. Remember that most of us have collaborated in this with our mutual funds, which we planned on having there for retirement.
- Pay-as-you-go approach. As expenses for benefits increase, the burden is placed on fewer employees. In time, this system will fall of its own accord if health care economics continue as they are.

We have all, though some more than others, been selfish in contributing to the ticking of this time bomb. The pendulum has swung too far toward the cold and calculating focus on money, and we are now seeing the consequences. The media may tell us daily that the financial economy, the stock market, is doing quite well, but the real economy, as seen in the breakdown of cities and communities because of health care expenses, is not doing well.

There is still huge denial regarding our health care crisis. This denial is shared by millions of individuals who choose to ignore how their lifestyle habits lead to symptoms of illness and by businesses and governments whose accounting practices permit them to hide the real costs of health care. There are many ways we have collectively created sleight of accounting in order to hide the real costs from ourselves.

Families in Sickness and Debt

It is becoming more obvious that low-income workers are suffering most in this health care meltdown. As reported in the *Arizona Republic* (January 18, 2006) only one-fourth of low-income people younger than sixty-five have job-based health insurance, compared to three-fourths of high-income people older than sixty-five. Many people must choose between paying rent and going to a doctor. As a result, more low-income people are driven onto the public Medicaid and Medicare programs. As long as this system is based on conventional allopathic medicine, it will fail economically and in healing. Furthermore, as many have experienced, being on such public programs can be humiliating.

Medicare

In the past two years, Medicare has essentially been converted into a feeding frenzy for pharmaceutical companies and insurance companies. From the simplicity of original Medicare, we now have a myriad of confusing programs, all carried out by private insurance firms that are more committed to stockholders than to patients, in spite of the rhetoric. Many elderly people, among others, know this, but feel helpless to do anything about it. This complexity in what was once simple and the overdependence on pharmaceuticals, hospitalizations, and procedures are costing us dearly and generating much fear—fear of illness, fear of going broke to pay for health care, fear of losing one's home. These factors will make Medicare increasingly financially unmanageable in coming years. It is important to recognize, in addition to the financial realities, that programs that generate unnecessary complexity and fear have as their hidden intent the control of people, rather than the creation of freedom. This is true, in spite of all rhetoric to the contrary.

Our current Medicare Drug Plan has two major problems:

1. It takes enrollees from a simple plan to something that is complex and confusing.
2. It makes the serious false assumption that almost exclusive use of pharmaceuticals means good health. This is a basic fallacy in health care today and, until corrected, will take us the wrong way economically and in healing.

Employer-Based Health Care Insurance

This is an area that is also melting down. Employers are feeling the increasing financial burden of health insurance for employees. Employees are feeling stress at the prospect of leaving a job that provides such insurance or in finding a job that includes this important benefit. And yet there is much resistance to changing the status quo. This resistance is present because of the hidden accounting practice built into employer-based insurance, which gives tax breaks to middle and higher income families when they buy health insurance through work. This may seem to be a good thing, but it is actually creating an increasing complexity that is confusing to both employer and employee.

In addition, there are other significant hidden aspects of this employer-based health insurance scheme. For example, even though the federal government provides $130 billion for Americans to buy health insurance, which is eleven percent of federal income tax revenue, this money is made available, not directly, but indirectly, through tax breaks to workers. In other words, we can receive health insurance from employers without having to pay income tax on its costs because the federal government is picking up the tab (Eduardo Porter, "Health Care for All, Just a Big Step Away," *New York Times*, December 18, 2005).

The problem with this subsidy, however noble it may seem, is that there is no way of accounting for it and identifying what it will and will not pay for. Without transparent accounting, these subsidies can be squandered by hidden people and organizations behind the scenes. Another problem with the hidden subsidy is who benefits from it. President Bush's advisory panel on tax reform reports that about half of this tax break or subsidy for health insurance accrues to families making more than $75,000 a year. More than a quarter goes to families making more than $100,000 a year. These families would surely hate to lose the subsidy. For a family making $100,000 a year in, say, Los Angeles, the tax break cuts the cost of employer-provided health insurance by about 35 percent in federal and state income taxes. In simple terms, a family making $100,000 per year saves $4,000 per year on health care insurance, and all taxpayers are picking up the tab for this without being informed. In summary, the subsidy goes to the people who need it less, those with more income, and it also encourages the wealthy to buy more insurance.

Part of the illusion today is that we think we can live separate lives and get away with it. We think we can go to work, make our money, buy what we want, have our real estate castle, make our future retirement funds out of the unearned income from rising speculative real estate values, and so on. These illusions are now being challenged. We all know we are all connected, or else there would not have been the great social contracts of the past half-century, contracts like Social Security and Medicare. Yet we are slow in awakening to the fact that these social contracts are falling apart, both in the business world and in the government sector.

In addition to this economic meltdown in health care that is affecting broad swaths of our society, there is the fact that the type of health care we think we need—essentially, pharmaceutical and hospital-based care—is increasingly ineffective in helping us to heal chronic illness and being able to afford such care. Whereas my book *Healthy Medicine* explored this in detail, we will look at this again from a more current financial perspective.

Chapter 2

HEALTH CARE 2006

HURRICANE KATRINA, THE hurricane that devastated New Orleans in 2005, was, in my view, a wake-up call. A clear message of this disaster was that we cannot afford to continue our practice of ignoring the inevitable until a disaster forces us to face it. In terms of health care, the approaching disaster is a catastrophic breakdown in the delivery of effective health care. If we do continue this practice, we face much higher financial and human costs of rebuilding the system, in addition to unnecessary devastating consequences to communities and people throughout the country.

The outlook for 2006 is an almost ten-percent increase in health care costs. This is more than triple the growth of general inflation. Under current demographics and health care organization, these costs will continue to rise in the years ahead The result is that more of these costs will be passed on to already financially overburdened workers and retirees. In twenty-eight percent of bankruptcies in 2005, the cause was debts from illness or injury. Annually, 400,000 families go bankrupt due to medical expenses. This is the population equivalent of a city the size of Albuquerque, New Mexico. The middle class is the most affected by this crisis.

In late 2005, two Wal-Mart memos came to light about ridding the company of employees who would cost what company executives considered too much in health care benefits. One of the memos described how forty-six percent of children of Wal-Mart employees are on Medicaid or uninsured.

The Wal-Mart memo exemplifies the views that many businesses across the country hold regarding health and employees. The following subjects were covered in the memo (my comments are in parentheses). The memo described how:

- Workers overuse emergency departments and underutilize prescriptions. (This overuse of ERs is common among the general population, for many reasons.)
- The least healthy employees want to work the longest in years. (Perhaps this is due to fear of the economic consequences of chronic illness.)
- The weak and sick are discouraged from seeking jobs. (This further erodes the trust that must be present between employer and employee; mistrust is now widespread.)
- Thirty-eight percent of workers spent one-sixth of their income on health care.

Unfortunately, as we will see in the coming pages, if the type of health care that employees' insurance policies cover or that they pay for themselves remains allopathic and pharmaceutical, health quality and chronic illness will worsen. It is time that we changed these societal rules, so that warmth of heart and enthusiasm tempers cold logic. This is what *Healthy Medicine* and *Beyond the Medical Meltdown* are all about.

Permit me to be direct. Where we are headed, if we continue on our current path of denial, is to the following:

- Sicker people with more severe and debilitating illnesses.
- Less insurance coverage or governmental help.
- More debt, bankruptcies, and home losses from such illnesses.
- Psychological stresses from the illnesses and their economic consequences.
- An epidemic of fear.

The responsibility for these situations is broad-based. The purpose of this book is not to crucify business or government. Individual denial and illness-generating lifestyles are epidemic. Each of us has our own responsibility to change our habits so that our lives can become healthier. The ways to do this are described in considerable detail in *Healthy Medicine* and I will not enlarge upon them here.

So how did we get into this predicament? Without clearly understanding this, we will not be able to move through it to the other side. Throughout this book, the reader will note a focus on the definition of good health care: effectiveness and affordability. In examining these two areas, we will come to understand why we are in crisis in health care and health care economics, and what steps we need to take to emerge from this crisis.

The Economy of Health

Let us look in detail at why health care costs are so high. Some of the main reasons today are:

- Overdependence on modern allopathic medicine: High-tech hospitals and pharmaceuticals.
- Bureaucracy and paperwork from a confusing multitude of private insurance companies, each looking for its place in the market.
- Risk of malpractice lawsuits, for a number of reasons discussed in *Healthy Medicine,* including a widespread societal tendency to look for scapegoats and pass the buck, in conjunction with the pervasive greed of the sickness care industry.
- Hidden tax subsidies and accounting practices, which have created a culture of understated hidden liabilities and overstated assets.

However some would prefer, the health care economy does not exist separate from the economy as a whole. Author Wendell Berry spoke to this in his suggestions for addressing change: Address the whole first. Piecemeal, one-shot solutions will not work.

Addressing the whole is the modus operandi of comprehensive medicine.

As economist Christopher Budd has described, what we have now is an economy that is more of a machine for making money, for private gain, something to be mined rather than something to be served and kept healthy.

Most of us are participating in this system. We have agreed to be a part of an economy in which our main purpose is to make money and amass possessions, for ourselves and for those close to us. Our quandary in health care is similar to the quandary in our economy as a whole. Just as we hope to hit the jackpot, in the lottery or some other way to make enough money so that we can retire early and have fun, we look for the quick fix for our illness symptoms.

It is out of this terrain that the morass of private insurance companies and other health care corporations have evolved, and continue to thrive and manipulate the "free market." They are not separate from us. They are not the bogeyman. The financing of medicine has become our master, not our servant. Is it more than a coincidence that we have exponential rises in cancer that accompany exponential rises in health care costs, as well as exponential rises in home prices? If our main income comes from non-earned income, what are we producing that has real value? We have all participated in seeking profit for profit's sake, and the consequences of this are now facing us in the health care meltdown, pension bailouts, and other crisis points in the news.

Historically, we humans have tended to place other people in authority over us. Once it was the priests in the ancient temples, then the kings and monarchs, and now the bankers, doctors, and corporate leaders. This has helped us to a certain degree. Witness especially the past 50 years of incredible growth in personal wealth, and even in the upgrading of social services for those at or near the bottom economically. But the consequences of giving our authority over to external authorities are now becoming apparent.

As a result of generations of giving our authority over to others, who today are the experts, we have what is called a top-down economy, and a top-down health care system. This means the control over our health is in the hands of others: doctors, insurance companies, governments, hospitals. Giving over our authority has led to overly expensive and ineffective healing of chronic illness, and to an expensive and bloated private health insurance bureaucracy. It has encouraged dependency, ignorance, and passivity in the face of authorities.

Therefore, out of this terrain of profit for the sake of profit, a terrain we have all collectively created and agreed on, we have:

- A health care system that is ill, because it has become primarily an industry.
- A deep fear and lack of trust in those we have assumed would have our best of health as their goal.
- A mutual denial by all parties in health care. I describe this in *Healthy Medicine.* It is based on the agreement between all parties that if the doctors and allied medical industries give therapies that eliminate symptoms, they will get paid. And the patient can therefore live in denial by thinking that the elimination of symptoms is the same as healing. It is not.

Health care has become primarily a commodity. A Hopi elder has referred to the casinos on Native American land as the commodification of the sacred. What this reflects is the extreme of "all individual and no society." As a result, we see most people today locked up in themselves, "caught between the tension of ever-increasing superficiality of a financial economy and ever-more sustenance conditions of the real economy," as Christopher Budd writes in *Rare Albion* (available through www.steinerbooks.org).

The problem is not money. Money is not the root of all evil. Some people have gone to the other extreme, blaming capitalism, wanting to wrest money away from the corporations and looking to government to take responsibility. But this is just another handing over of authority, and no longer suffices in solving today's critical problems.

There is a third way, a middle way, which we will explore as this book progresses. Before doing this, however, we must further examine and clearly understand what has happened to health care.

Myth and Reality

Myth: The United States has the best health care system in the world.

Reality: The United States has the most overpriced health care system in the world, one that furthers disease rather than supporting healing. For the most part, our health care system causes disease rather than healing it. Some reports are now that, "medical tourism," Americans seeking good health care abroad, is growing dramatically. The U.S. health care system has been rated a poor seventy-second worldwide. The myth is an illusion based on patriotic pride.

Myth: Scientific breakthroughs will liberate us from illness and end human suffering.

Reality: Modern medicine with its greed and its mechanistic approaches only shifts the suffering from one part of the body to another or one person to another. These approaches lead to more fear and dependency, and more profits from the illness and suffering of others.

Myth: There are fast and easy cures that can solve our health problems.

Reality: Healing requires time, patience, insight, lifestyle changes, and the assistance of perceptive and compassionate practitioners who can guide us through the layers of illness that most of us have in our lives.

Myth: All infectious diseases will be eradicated.

Reality: Bugs are smart; they exchange genetic information and build resistance to our drugs, especially antibiotics.

Myth: "The private sector always works better in the marketplace than government." (This was a statement made by Republican Rep. Doug Quelland of Arizona, as reported in the *Arizona Republic* [January 20, 2006].)

Reality: The private sector, through its excessive greed, its health care bureaucracy that is far larger than that of government, and its tremendously confusing and fragmented insurance care system, is not, in its present state, any better than government in the health care marketplace. Corporate handlers in insurance, pharmaceutical companies and hospitals now dictate to the marketplace what will and will not be covered under a given insurance policy. They dictate the type of medical practice that is acceptable —those approved by medical boards. The original charter of corporations is that they exist for enhancing the common good. This fact has been lost and must be resurrected.

Myth: If we bring more people under the insurance umbrella, then health care will become more affordable.

Reality: The present health insurance model, with its many flaws described in these pages, cannot help us anymore. We must remove the umbrella and create new forms of health care associations and practice.

The result of these perpetuated myths and illusions is fear of illness, fear of financial devastation from the costs of care for illness, and fear that our caretakers are more focused on furthering their own profit situation rather than on our health and well-being. Any change in health care must address these deep imbalances and change them fundamentally. This will require big changes for everyone.

An increasing number of people have already begun to see through these myths and illusions. For example, we know that the promise of antibiotics has not been borne out. The arrogance apparent in these myths is still pervasive in the medical field, however. The challenge to medicine today is to find applicants with the wisdom of the heart to accompany their intellectual abilities, and then not brainwash them in four years of medical school, but rather educate them in both conventional and alternative medicine, and cultivate tolerance and receptivity to many approaches to healing.

The problems in current health care thinking, with an overemphasis on often unnecessary, ineffective, and increasingly expensive diagnostic and treatment methods, derive from two core issues: these methods are primarily allopathic and specialty oriented, and distant, cold third parties determine when they will be used.

The first issue, that these methods of diagnosis and treatment are primarily allopathic, is a huge hypnotism that it will be necessary to break in the coming years if we are to heal individually and economically. This illusion is shattering as more Americans wake up. There has not been, however, much more than a trickle of real change in corporate boardrooms and government halls. As stated earlier, conventional or allopathic medicine has come to be seen as normal and good. We accept such things as antibiotics and other drugs, vaccines, CT scans, surgery, and cardiac catheterizations as being what health care is all about. We, both patients and medical professionals, think of the use of these drugs and procedures as normal and good because we tell ourselves that:

- "They get rid of symptoms."
- "Someone else will pay for them."
- "Everyone does it, so it must be right."
- "My job and the jobs of many others depend on this medicine."

The reality is that our tremendous overdependence on allopathic specialty medicine has made significant dents in our quality of care and our economics. Access to such care is declining among Medicaid patients and the uninsured. It is more expensive and restrictive among the insured. It is more available to the chronically ill Medicare patient, not because it is more effective but because it is built into Medicare laws, and because these patients do not have to pay the bill, though this is changing.

The fear of not being able to see a specialist is rampant. Those who benefit from allopathic care continuing to be the primary model encourage this fear. Yet specialty high-tech care does not lead to greater healing. It treats you as a machine with disconnected parts. (*Healthy Medicine* discusses why these allopathic approaches are predominant) The reality is that high-tech specialty care must become an ever-smaller part of health care if we are to create a more balanced and healthy medical system. We must come to see the reality that the methods of allopathic medicine have valuable but limited capacity to help us heal.

Corporate Health Care

A primary subject in both this book and *Healthy Medicine* is individual responsibility in self-care and professional responsibility to be more open to all modes of therapy. This section looks at the role of the corporate world in medicine. Let me say, again, that I am not approaching this discussion with the attitude that corporations are bad. The greed with which the corporate world now engages in the health care industry is only reflective of our national imbalance, but it nevertheless feeds it and needs to change if health care is to become both effective and affordable.

After looking at corporate influence in health care, we will move on to health insurance. Then *Beyond the Medical Meltdown* will turn to discussion of what we can constructively do to change our approach.

Today, corporations in health care include insurance companies, pharmaceuticals, hospitals, medical and surgical supply companies, and many physician practices. The mandate of the corporation is to protect the shareholder's investment. The question today is how this mandate is balanced with respect to the health care service for which the corporation is responsible. Today, most corporations have no bounds in the pursuit of self-interest. And they have less and less accountability for damage to third parties, whether those third parties are local communities, the environment, or consumers.

American business today is based on the corporation, as is most business in the world. What is a corporation? It is not a person. Because it is not a person, it has no personal hope. It is basically a pile of money. It does not age. It goes about its business as if it is immortal. "Its single purpose: accumulate more money" (Wendell Berry, *The Presence of Fear*). Because a corporation as an entity has no remorse, it cannot feel like humans feel, and so suffers no regret regarding the negative effects of its actions on our children and grandchildren.

This book is not suggesting the banning of corporations. When run correctly, corporations can be effective vehicles for service. The goal of corporations in health care needs to change from protecting the stockholder's investment to serving the healing of people. The reality is that if we focus on the second, the first can also happen. Serving the healing process in people means local hospitals offering comprehensive medicine and a local, decentralized practitioner economy of health care. Capital ownership of health care institutions, technology, and products has a social responsibility that is largely ignored today.

The next chapter explores the changes necessary. Suffice it to say here that with this transformation of health care, with insurance policies that permit people the freedom to choose their own practitioner (M.D. or otherwise), with both personal and corporate responsibility built into such a new system, the result will be a community enriched and a people with ample tools to heal.

The High Price of Overdependence on Allopathic Medicine

Earlier, I mentioned some of the main causes of the high price of health care today. This included such important areas as overdependence on pharmaceuticals and the other main therapies and diagnostic procedures of allopathic medicine. Here, I discuss this further.

The bureaucracy and the legal malpractice situation have grown out of health care's reliance on pharmaceuticals, hospitalization, and expensive medical procedures and supplies.

1. PHARMACEUTICALS

Today, our half-century addiction to pharmaceuticals is stronger than ever. The new Medicare law will build this into our government financing even more than now. The barrage of pharmaceutical commercials on television creates hypnosis. Advertisers know that when exposed to something enough, people tune it out consciously, and yet the message then goes into the subconscious and motivates behavior. This mental manipulation is widespread today.

Pharmaceutical "normalcy" is supported by such methods as:

- Aggressive marketing with direct to the public ads.
- Bribing doctors to prescribe, and calling these "consulting fees."
- Promoting fraudulent "scientific" drug trials.
- Markups of up to 500,000 percent on some prescription drugs.

In *Overdo$ed America,* Dr. John Abramson states that $570 billion per year in medicine is spent on drugs that are harmful or not effective. The U.S. Food and Drug Administration (FDA) is deeply involved with making sure this pharmaceutical normalcy continues, in spite of the rhetoric that it protects the public. Such FDA practices as rapid approval of inadequately tested drugs, focus on discrediting herbs, and attempts to over-regulate nutritional supplements illustrate this. Whereas there are a number of herbs and supplements on the market that are not good quality, such substances have a tiny fraction, if any at all, of the side effects of drugs.

Phrases heard today that are subtly meant to convince us that pharmaceutical drugs are safe include:

- "Tried and true."
- "Most drugs work."
- "More research is needed."

The response to these phrases, from a comprehensive medicine perspective, is:

- "Tried and true" applies to many non-allopathic therapies that are well proven to be effective and affordable in helping us to heal.

- Most drugs work on a chemical level to make changes in us, yet these changes more often than not create many more problems than they help. The recent Vioxx case, which revealed significant cardiovascular side effects from this drug prescribed for osteoarthritis, pain, rheumatoid arthritis, and migraines, is but one of many examples that these changes are often known years before a drug is released, and yet the results are suppressed by the manufacturer.

- The phrase "more research is needed" is meant to suppress the sale of any product that does not have millions of dollars of research and clinical trials to back it up. The only companies that can afford such research are the pharmaceutical corporations. Much smaller companies that make very good and effective products that, for example, improve heart function much better than does a cholesterol-lowering drug, are shut out of the insurance market because of these built-in hypnotic phrases. The same is true now in agriculture, where small organic farms can no longer afford to spend the large amounts of money to be certified organic, because larger farms have influenced the passage of laws that favor them over the smaller farms.

But are pharmaceutical drugs necessary? More than 100,000 deaths per year are due to misuse of pharmaceuticals. Yet it makes headline news when one person dies from using an herb along with a prescribed drug. This is how distorted the media is.

The side effects of drugs are increasing. Television commercials for various drugs reel off myriad side effects (drug companies are required to disclose these in advertisements), but they are often cited so quickly that we cannot hear them, and said as voiceover to images of happy people.

The plain truth is that pharmaceuticals, for the most part, do not help us heal. They work on specific biochemical levels to alter our symptoms so that we are more comfortable. But they do not induce the increased tissue oxygenation, enhanced cell function, and improved organ function that support real healing, as many comprehensive medicine therapies do.

In the book *Generation Rx*, author Greg Critser states that pharmaceutical companies have achieved the following objectives:

- Coopted the federal government.
- Seduced the medical establishment.
- Mesmerized the public.
- Convinced everyone that regulations are harmful.

America is obsessed and hypnotized with the belief that drugs help us heal. Unless this hypnotism is broken, the influence of pharmaceuticals on our medical system will grow stronger, with disastrous results for people's health and the economic well-being of individuals and communities.

2. HOSPITALS

There is a hospital building boom, especially in the suburbs. An article in *USA Today* (Dennis Cauchon and Julie Appleby, "Hospital Building in the Burbs," January 3, 2006) called this a development that is expected to "increase the use of high-tech medicine and add fuel to rising health care costs." Then why do we do this? In this author's perception, there are three main reasons:

1. We still are under the hypnosis that high-tech = better health.
2. Corporate health care is able to create demand through advertising and through control of health insurance payments.
3. It is still ethical to invest even when there is not a need.

This last point deserves consideration. Part of the ethos of extreme capitalism is that corporations make investments even when there is not a need. Of course the question becomes, who decides the need, and also, whose need? Who decides if the expense to the average person, and to the health of local and national economy, is worth the expenditure? The answer is that these decisions are now being made, in health care and in many other areas of life in the United States, by fewer and fewer people and corporations. We can see this in the sell-off of public utilities to a few private interests, in the sell-off of public schools to private interests, in the prison system, and also, of course, in health care.

In this hospital boom, we see more suburban hospitals, because this is where the money is, not necessarily where the need is. The suburbs are where the best-insured people live. We see more expensive and luxurious buildings with profitable treatments, especially those in cardiovascular, cancer, and neonatal care. The *USA Today* article quotes Dr. John Wennberg, director of the Center for Evaluative Clinical Sciences at Dartmouth Medical School: "These hospitals are loaded with technology to intensively treat chronically ill patients right up to death."

This is an important comment. It means that the growth in health care expenses, local jobs, and stock-market portfolios depends on there being an increase in what one author has called a "feeder system" of chronically ill patients. It means that the survival of our entire health care system depends on having an increasing number of chronically ill patients. Do you, reader, want to be one of these people? Do you want someone in your family or business or circle of friends to be one of the people in this feeder system?

This is the same as having local and state economies depend on tobacco companies being able to sell more cigarettes, even if it is to people overseas (that is their problem, so it goes), and depending on casinos staying in business even if this does not produce any real products for communities.

These hospital booms are going on in cities all over the country. In Indianapolis, there are four new heart-surgery centers, as well as an orthopedic hospital, all built since 2004. These employ a lot of people, support the local tax base, and give people money to spend. But at what price? I refer the reader to *The Last Well Person: How to Stay Well Despite the Health-Care System,* by Nortin M. Hadler, M.D., professor of medicine at the University of North Carolina Medical School. He and other doctors are criticizing the current trend of performing more and more cardiovascular stents and surgeries.

We must find a way to bring common sense back into these health care financing equations. For example, if I have chest pain, why does it cost so much to go the ER and have an EKG and blood tests? Why does an ER doctor make $150 per hour? Why are the other expenses so high? Why have I not had a much less expensive cardiovascular evaluation and individualized low-tech comprehensive medical treatments before now?

Why are my biochemistry, physiology, and immune system not being monitored for functional abnormalities that precede cancer and other chronic diseases?

We can no longer afford to have thousands of people undergo endoscopies of the stomach, at $900 a procedure, to look for causes of illness, before treating the condition with much less expensive and often effective methods of which most so-called alternative medical practitioners are well aware.

Who decides the costs of these expensive allopathic procedures, relative to other costs? Who decides that a preventative treatment for diabetic foot problems with a podiatrist, for $200, is not to be reimbursed by insurance, but a $10,000 foot amputation as a result of lack of good podiatric care is.

Many practitioners of comprehensive or integrative medicine already know that many expensive surgeries are unnecessary and can be prevented. Yet these experiences are not considered at all in the decisions about whether to build hospitals or to promote the latest cholesterol-lowering drugs. This points to the lack of ethics in our health care decision-making corporations, and a lack of inclusiveness. These are characteristic of a system gone out of balance to the extreme, the extreme edge of capitalism, which is a system that, when operating in a balanced way, is a good system of economics.

We need to evolve beyond this, so that it becomes the social norm to invest only when there is a need for investment. Again, the primary purpose of health care and of economy in general is to serve human needs and creativity. So are our needs served by the trend of building more hospitals and needing more chronically ill people to keep the system making ever more profits? Many, including this author, would suggest that the answer is no.

The fact that a corporation, or an individual, can borrow money in order to do something is neither proof of the need for that thing nor justification for its production. Currently, our social norm is that it is right to do something just because it can be done, or just because we can borrow the money to do so. Again, who is responsible for these decisions? Who is responsible for our economic lives?

Our taxes pay for 46 percent of the nation's medical care, mostly through Medicare and Medicaid, the costs of both of which are bankrupting local economies nationwide and worsening the health of elderly and disabled people through an increase in pharmaceutical treatments provided by the Medicare Law of 2003. Yet even though almost half of these expenses are borne by everyone, the hospitals, especially the glut of for-profit hospitals, are beholden to stockholders, not the general public that pays taxes. This does not make sense.

A director of one of these for-profit hospitals stated, "I look at the busted bones and old hips, and heart disease in old guys like me. I have to say, demand looks pretty good." Until enough people see through this preposterous way of doing health care, and become more actively involved in changing this, things will continue and the health of most Americans will worsen, and local economies will suffer more.

3. MEDICAL PROCEDURES AND SUPPLIES

We have a similar situation today with hospital procedures as we have with drugs. In *The Last Well Person,* Dr. Hadler states that "bypass surgery belongs in the medical archives." Virtually daily now, the news exposes more corruption and dishonesty portraying itself as medical science at the highest levels of pharmaceutical and hospital supply companies.

No health care reform will be successful in providing both effective and affordable health care for all without making major changes in the financing of three areas of health care: interventional cardiology, that is, bypass surgeries, stents, and complex diagnostic procedures; pharmaceuticals in cancer care; and end-of-life heroics.

INTERVENTIONAL CARDIOLOGY

As Dr. Hadler states, there are far too many cardiac procedures being done in the United States, many more than are actually needed. The statistics today are that more than 500,000 cardiac bypass graft surgeries are performed per year and more than 650,000 coronary angioplasties per year, at a total cost of $25 billion annually. Local economies throughout the country have come to depend on these surgeries being performed, so that cities increase their tax revenues and more people are employed. These procedures support almost every hospital in the United States.

The question is: who decides whether such a procedure will be performed? Is the cardiac physician today an impartial observer, the champion of his or her patient's health and well-being? Of course cities need income and people need work, but if the mechanism to supply the income and jobs is built into health care, these procedures are assumed as necessary, with statements like, "That's just the way it is."

Who decides if these extremely expensive procedures are needed for health? As long as we do not have impartial observers, referees if you will, then the so-called private health care medical-industrial complex will make these decisions, continue to do many more of these procedures than are called for, and further drive up health care costs. There is much good research in integrative medicine that there are ways through lifestyle changes, nutrition, supplements, and other programs to heal heart disease without such expensive medical procedures. If we want to curtail these procedures, we must at the same time lower people's expectations for receiving them. As it is, with their expectations raised, people tend to see any attempt to curtail them as government rationing.

Pharmaceutical Therapies in Cancer

The use of chemotherapy as a first-line therapy in cancer does not make sense. In spite of more than 30 years of the war on cancer, there is no convincing evidence that these therapies have made much of a dent in improving survival in cancer. Furthermore, the new generation of cancer drugs, some of which have hardly had the necessary time for in-depth study of effectiveness, are already being commonly used. The cost-benefit analysis: These drugs can cost more than $200,000 per patient, for an extension of life of up to 14 months, and with the suffering involved with chemotherapy and end-stage cancer.

Again, we must ask, who decides? What most of the public does not know, because of media suppression and the rigid thinking, hidden financial motivations, and desire to stay in control that characterize allopathic medicine today, is that there are many well-proven so-called alternative medicine therapies for cancer. To learn about these, I refer the reader to *The Moss Reports* (customized reports by Dr. Ralph Moss, available at www.cancerdecisions.com). The $200,000 that it costs to treat one person with the new cancer drugs could help many patients to heal cancer with a more comprehensive and inclusive medical approach, which could involve the judicious use of low doses of chemotherapy combined with other alternative therapies.

End-of-life Therapies

It is well known that much of the rising costs in health care today go toward keeping people alive and on respirators for days to weeks beyond the natural time that they might die. This approach is built into medicine now. It has legal safeguards and protections for the hospitals and doctors who continue this, often for mixed motives. These motives include:

- A belief in medicine that letting a patient die means the doctor has not done his or her job.
- Money: Hospitals make enormous amounts of money by continuing this often barbaric practice.
- Inertia and routine: "This is just how it is done today."
- Fear of lawsuits: Because families often demand this care, doctors and hospitals legitimately continue this practice.

So the rise in these health care costs, which surely will grow as the population ages, can be attributed to the massive collusion and denial of everyone involved. The question becomes: Who can stop or significantly curtail the practice of prolonging life? Neither the medical profession nor hospitals nor families nor lawyers want it to stop. It will take a public forum. Stopping or curtailing it is a public responsibility.

If we approach this with common sense, and observe clearly, we can see that most people at this stage of life do not want to go through this, that most often these approaches are not successful other than for a few days or weeks, and that most families want this to happen not because their loved ones who are dying want it, but because family members do not want to let go.

Who Decides?

This is an area I address in *Healthy Medicine*. But it is an important issue, so I will discuss it here also.

Currently, decisions about health care are most often made by doctors, hospitals, and insurance company representatives. The problem with this arrangement is that both parties are increasingly influenced by the financial motivations of medical corporations with their stockholders. The patient is most often not involved in this process. Patients are expected to be what I call DIPs—dependent, ignorant, and passive.

In addition, the concept of P4P, or pay for performance, is entering into health care decisions. The idea with this is that insurance companies reward health care providers that meet certain cost, quality, and patient satisfaction goals. The problems here are in such questions as, who determines quality of care and what if the patient stays in denial and does not change his or her life, as in quitting smoking. Performance-based models may work for fixing cars, but not people.

The issue of who decides needs to become a collaborative decision-making process between doctor and patient. In this arrangement, however, both doctor and patient are different from what they are today. The doctor is a free agent whose primary role here is the best health of the patient, and the patient is active, involved, willing to make lifestyle changes, co-responsible. The big unknown here is insurance companies, which the next section addresses.

On what basis health care decisions are made is related to who makes the decision. Asking and answering the following questions can provide some guidelines for decision-making:

- How do we determine cost-effectiveness?
- How do we determine whether a therapy is effective?
- Are there objective witnesses anymore who are not invested in a particular answer coming out of a study?

Today, there are three essential ways to determine effectiveness:

- Double-blind studies: This research model is the so-called "tried and true" method that modern, "scientific" medicine puts forth as the only legitimate model. Such studies are often, however, a scam of false science and influenced by assumptions that rule our health care today. Double-blind research often requires millions of dollars. This means, in effect, that the only therapies that will be approved in hospitals and insurance companies are pharmaceutical and medical technology therapies that are backed by big money.

- Evidence-based studies: This type of research is also used by conventional medicine and increasingly by integrative medicine. It is based on the objective evidence of a clinical trial.
- Results-based studies: These are what modern medicine often derisively calls "anecdotal" or "unproven" studies. It is often out of these studies, however, that very good therapies are developed. We need a health care system that incorporates such research into our decision-making.

Health Insurance

Now let us look at the whole area of health insurance. When it comes to health insurance, what people today want to know are the answers to three questions:

1. How will I be able to afford the health care I need?
2. What will my money buy me in health care?
3. Will I be able to go to the doctor I want?

1. How will I be able to afford the health care I need?

Most people are under increasing financial stress. This can be seen in:

- Less savings.
- Higher household debt.
- More work hours per week for less pay.
- Breakdown of family matrix with less time at home.
- Bankruptcies from health care expenses rising significantly.

2. WHAT WILL MY MONEY BUY ME IN HEALTH CARE?

Providing an answer to this is becoming more difficult. Witness the confusion that most Medicare-eligible people are now experiencing because of the 2003 Medicare law that is to go into effect in 2006. Those with private insurance often experience the same frustrations, with myriad policies and fine-print qualifications.

3. WILL I BE ABLE TO GO TO THE DOCTOR I WANT?

Due to the current complicated health care insurance system that we have created in the belief that the market knows best, even in its chaos, most people are not able to work with their doctor of choice. They are assigned to a doctor or they cannot leave their assigned doctor if they do not like him or her. It is important for people to be able to choose their doctor. This is not only true for the obvious reasons of rights to freedom of choice. It is also true for healing. When we are working with our practitioner of choice, a healing energy is generated between patient and doctor. This is based on trust, which can help heal the many fears that accompany illness.

The insurance industry is not focused on answering these three questions to the satisfaction of most people. The insurance industry is an industry. This fact is an important sign of how we have commodified health care. The focus of health insurance companies is: How can our company collect more premiums and pay out less in expenses for care for enrollees?

This sets up an adversarial relationship. Let us be clear here. Adversarial relationships are not necessarily bad. When we were all growing up, we often perceived our parents as adversaries when they told us we could not have something we wanted. We needed someone with greater wisdom and experience than we had to set some boundaries for us. We also need this as adults, since most of us have not successfully worked through some of these childhood issues. Most people are still in denial about the extent of their illness-generating lifestyle habits, and these illness-generating lifestyle habits are the results of denial, so it is a vicious circle. The difference between the parental relationship and that of the insurance company, however, is that our parents cared for us, for our health and well-being. They did not see us as adversaries. Health insurance companies do see us as adversaries, regardless of the message they communicate in their advertisements.

Detrimental adversarial relationships now exist between doctors and patients, between doctors and hospitals, and between patients and insurance companies. One result is fear among the general public: fear of illness and its suffering, fear of the cost of illness, and fear of losing one's job.

Health insurance is a good idea gone astray. In the past, this insurance covered most expenses. Today, due to a number of reasons—technology, greed, lack of healthy lifestyles, toxic environments, to name a few—the cost of health insurance is becoming a heavier and heavier drag on the economy.

Remember that health insurance companies' reason for existence is to reward stockholders. Are you, the reader, a stockholder in an insurance company? Does your portfolio include mutual funds that are invested in health insurance companies? If so, then you are trying to play both ends. You want the best of health care and you want your insurance company to pay for whatever health care needs you and your family have. Yet you also want increasing dividends from your stock portfolio. This means that the health insurance companies must pay out as little as possible to their patients, so that you can make more money. Obviously, there is a conflict here. We must work to resolve this conflict so that each of us can receive the health care we need and still have enough money to live on. But this is another built-in conflict in our economy that we choose to deny. The bill is now due for this denial.

Health insurance companies today focus on youth-oriented insurance. We see slick marketing catering to populations they hope are ignorant of these issues, so they can skim off the young and healthy. The market has now brought us to a survival-of-the-fittest state of health care. The result is low-risk people with lousy health insurance and high-risk people who are unable to afford health care. The reason is higher deductibles, higher co-payments, and higher premiums, which is what most people are now experiencing as a result of insurance company efforts to shift blame, shift paperwork, and find someone else to foot the bill.

The state of mind behind these efforts is commonplace not only in insurance companies and government circles, but also in the general population. The Mercer National Survey of Employer-sponsored Health Plans 2005 reports that there is a "new willingness on the part of employers—born of desperation" to shift the cost to their employees. This creates an adversarial relationship between worker and employer and a system based on fear and control. Employers increasingly perceive their employees as a financial liability they have to endure in order to produce a product or service. Employers are worried about their businesses being viable, and employees are fearful of not having jobs and income.

The cost-shifting approaches of employers regarding health care include:

• Increasing the percentage of premiums paid by the employee.
• Raising the deductibles and co-payments of employees.
• Increasing the cost-sharing in other ways.
• Limiting workers' choices of insurance plans.

I must reiterate here that the purpose of this writing is not to demonize health insurance companies. They are only doing what we have given them license to do: make a profit, at our expense and due to our denial. Also, be mindful that much of the population still eats at fast-food restaurants, doesn't exercise, uses illegal drugs or legal stimulants, stays up late and gets up early—and the list of our imbalances goes on. So each of us has a responsibility for our collective health care dilemma.

This being said, we have created a health insurance scheme in which:

- Investors and stockholders are valued over patient care and over employee well-being.
- Only conventional medicine diagnostic and therapeutic interventions are reimbursed. This is creating huge economic problems.
- Preexisting conditions severely restrict people's capacity to find the health care they need. The reality is that all illnesses are preexisting. Illness that appears in one's fifties almost always has its origin in very early life, and in the subsequent lifestyle imbalances that grew out of these early life experiences.

To not insure patients because they had some chest pain or headaches ten years earlier sends the message to all people that their symptoms are a liability to the very people they are paying to help them when they are ill. It also creates an environment where a person has to lie and cover up prior symptoms in order to purchase insurance.

Today, there are an increasing number of part-time workers with low-wage jobs with no health insurance. This means no protection against the tremendously and artificially inflated "free market" in health care. Many of these people want federal and state government to step in and pay for health insurance. But what if there are no government surpluses to pay for these services? What if the type of health care insurance that government would underwrite for insurance companies is ineffective in many cases of chronic illness and far too expensive because of its ineffectiveness? What if insurance companies, guaranteed government backing, increase restrictions and refuse coverage more frequently due to preexisting conditions.

Insurance Gambits

Preexisting conditions

Current: Many people are denied health care insurance because of preexisting conditions, or their insurance rates are greatly inflated, putting increased financial pressure on many families and individuals.

Reality: Everyone has preexisting conditions. Cancer takes one to two decades to develop into lesions large enough to be detected on X-rays or blood tests. Almost everyone in the United States today has lived for many years with the toxic load (from chemicals, heavy metals, microorganisms, and drugs), nutritional deficiencies, and organ dysfunctions that virtually guarantee the development of chronic heart disease, cancers, and/or neurological degenerative disorders at an ever earlier time in life.

The use of the preexisting condition rule in insurance rating is a scam, a means of controlling people, and a way of generating even more fear of the economic incapacitation of chronic illness

The only way around this is to: recognize and acknowledge the reality of preexisting conditions in everyone, and support people in healing these preconditions before they become deeper problems. This means expanding our health practices to include most of what is now called alternative medicine.

When a man reports in an application for insurance that he has occasional heartbeat irregularities, for example, instead of turning him down for insurance or demanding much higher premiums, co-pays, and deductibles, we must instead be happy we have discovered this problem in his life. We can be happy about this because, with comprehensive medicine, we know the ways to help this problem correct itself before pathological heart disease develops.

When we have this attitude, we create an environment of trust, not fear. The current economic environment of preexisting conditions in insurance applications generates fear of higher, incapacitating health care costs. By doing a 180 here, and changing directions on how we approach preexisting conditions, health care costs will fall and people's health will improve.

This will likely not be possible unless we make the change from insurance-controlled health care to associative-based health care. Insurance companies might still exist in such a system, but their role will be fundamentally different, as described later.

Before continuing, let us take a look at two trends that are growing as we enter 2006: health savings accounts and boutique practices.

HEALTH SAVINGS ACCOUNTS

With a health savings account, a person can have a high deductible for major medical insurance. There are more companies offering these. The individual accumulates money tax free, and can either spend it on medical services or save it to pay for future health care costs. The potential problem here is that these health savings accounts, or HSAs, will become tax shelters for those who are more affluent.

The use of health savings accounts has two significant ramifications. First, it creates the illusion that each of us can afford to pay for the care we will need to heal our illnesses. The great majority of people cannot. With the tremendous social irresponsibility of the past decades on the part of major corporations in industry, agriculture, and medicine that have lead to a plethora of environmentally related illnesses, these illnesses will not be cheap to heal. They will require time, energy, and effective comprehensive medicine therapies. These costs will have to be shared in some way.

Second, this type of financial arrangement will motivate many of those who can afford to have such health savings accounts to save the money and not spend the necessary funds on their health care. Out of fear, they will save for a rainy day rather than invest in health-promoting therapies. There is an idea here in health savings accounts that can be positive if restructured. This is the idea that individuals and families would have these accounts not to invest the savings, but rather to invest in effective and affordable health care.

Many businesses are looking to HSAs as a way to cut health care costs and shift more financial responsibility to employees. This once again pits employees against employers, both still caught in the web of market manipulation by corporate health care industry players—insurance companies, pharmaceutical companies, and hospitals, to name three.

Unfortunately, this movement toward HSAs is being deceptively promoted in a fashion similar to that of tax cuts: that HSAs will put more money and control in the hands of consumers. The HSA approach could be worthwhile, but only if consumers can freely choose the care they want, and only if the large corporate players discontinue manipulating behind the scenes through advertising, deceptive accounting practices, and government-pushed regulations that further weaken the consumer's real options.

What is contained in this movement toward HSAs is, however, an underlying effort to help businesses, especially small businesses, by lifting the burden of rising health care costs from their bottom line in order to improve profitability. This is a good idea if it is done right. Unfortunately, the way it is being done currently is not the right way, but rather just a continuance of market manipulation. Doing it right will mean moving away from employer-based financing of health care and toward health associations, as described in the next chapter. This, when combined with the principles of healthy medicine, will lower the costs and increase the quality of our health care.

Boutique Medicine

This is conventional medicine's answer to an impersonal medical system. It is an answer, again, for those with money. The key ingredient of this growing practice is that, for a yearly stipend of between $1,500 and $2,000, patients receive much more time and attention from their doctor. They also get the latest in electronic communications. One of the catchphrases today in health care reform talk is that, by upgrading computer communications, people receive better care. This is most likely just another smoke-and-mirrors approach to health care, high-tech glitz that covers up a conventional medical model that is increasingly ineffective in healing chronic illness.

In boutique practices, patients get quick referral to a specialist. Although seeing a surgeon or a cardiologist quickly can be lifesaving, such specialists are most often not needed. A good general practitioner of comprehensive medicine can treat most problems. This promise of referral to specialists is another appeal to peoples fears that if they do not see specialists they will not get well. It feeds a continued over-reliance on specialists, most of whom depend on expensive and far over-utilized diagnostic and therapeutic equipment.

The underlying problems with boutique medicine are:

- It is based on allopathy, a failed system in itself.
- It is indulgent to patient whims, with the promise by the doctor to be available 24/7 to any patient, and to refer to specialists whenever the patient wants. One must wonder how such a physician can be honest with the patient, for fear of losing income, when the physician must point out changes the patient needs to make in order to become healthier.
- It is financially unavailable to most people today.

Basically, boutique medicine is the response of allopathic medical doctors who want to continue practicing in the same way, using the same therapies, and want less interference in their work from government and insurance companies. This is the goal of most doctors, including those in alternative medicine. The problem is that it is an end run around the responsibility that the conventional medicine profession bears in having created our current complex insurance system.

There are both practitioners and patients who like boutique medicine. This is often because the doctor can spend more time with the patient. This is admirable and is a step in the right direction. But because it is still primarily allopathic, boutique medicine as it exists now cannot succeed in improving patient healing and cutting the costs of health care for society as a whole.

Why the Bush Health Care Agenda Will Fail

1. *The focus is primarily on containing costs.* This is a limited and mechanistic approach. If the primary practice of medicine remains allopathic, as it was in both the Clinton and Bush approaches, all efforts at cost control will fail, because the "free market" of modern high-tech pharmaceutical medicine will guarantee a rise in health care costs and a rationing of care, without calling it this.

2. *The Bush philosophy is to place more responsibility in the hands of individuals, ostensibly to create market pressure to hold down costs.* Placing more responsibility for their own health in the hands of individuals is, of course, necessary for any health care to become more effective. But this will not create market pressure to hold down costs. This is because the market interest of those who manipulate market forces from behind the scenes (i.e., pharmaceutical companies and specialty hospitals that have to have a certain number of patients wheeled into surgery and CT suites in order to survive financially) is not in the interests of health. Their market interest is in having a sicker population that is more dependent, more fearful, and more passive.

3. *The central focus of Bush proposals is tax breaks.* Both Democrat and Republican experts have said that this is likely to drive up rather than lower health care costs. Again, we have the seductive appeal of tax cuts being used to manipulate people into believing this will lower their health care costs. This is a wolf in sheep's clothing. Such proposals as expanding health savings accounts will primarily benefit people with higher incomes and more savings, and will be a multibillion-dollar boon to banks and investment companies.

A time is rapidly approaching for all Americans when we will have to ask ourselves what we are demanding in health care. We will have to pare back our demands, prune the tree of excess demands, cut to the essence of what really helps us. For this to happen, business leaders in large and small businesses will have to engage their employees in a new way. This is an associative way, as described in this book. Business too often perceives labor costs adversarially, as in the Wal-Mart memo regarding sick employees demonstrates. Employers need to enter into partnership with employees and discuss the impact of rising health care costs. In this way, employers and employees can see that it is in both their interests to come together and bargain for good health care. This is what will lower costs and improve individual health and the business's bottom line.

Interestingly, the Bush proposal for small businesses across the country to band together and buy health insurance has some potential, but only if small business owners realize they need to think out of the box. Both employers and employees need to see clearly that without collaborating in the spirit of mutual responsibility, without fundamentally changing the concept of "coverage" to include comprehensive medicine, and without applying sustainable wellness principles to make the work environment and home environment healthier, all efforts at controlling costs are doomed to fail, because people will become sicker.

If small businesses and individuals work together to remove control of health care from the big corporate players (insurance companies, pharmaceutical companies, hospitals, and medical supply companies) and decentralize health care into local control, and if they apply the main principles of healthy medicine, their efforts have a chance of succeeding.

In addition, Bush is correct in perceiving that current health care tax subsidies, in which employers who pay health insurance premiums for employees can deduct the payments as a business expense on their tax returns and the payments are not counted as taxable income for the employees, is indeed unfair to individuals who are seeking insurance. But Bush's answer to this perceived unfairness is to put the single individual at a further disadvantage in the present runaway greed of market forces that are not really interested in our health and well-being. The call for decreasing federal control and increasing patient control, in reality, puts all of us even more at the mercy of ruthless market forces. This increases fear and helplessness among individuals and small business owners. And this is what ruthless market forces want.

The Bush proposals purport to help the individual taxpayer, but they continue tax schemes that are really hidden subsidies, and permit the uninsured population to grow. The result will be that the health costs for all of us will rise, and the severity of chronic illness and its costs to quality of life and to communities will become more severe.

We do not have wiggle room anymore to "fix it in the mix." The Bush approaches are manipulative and superficial, and will permit the same so-called free-market forces in health care to continue to control and exploit health care, protected by new laws that give them freedom to manipulate without responsibility.

In concluding this chapter, it can be said that with "normal" conventional modern medicine and its economic arrangements, we now have:

- Impaired healing.
- Impaired economic security.
- Impaired freedom.

In answer to the question of what we need in health care, there are three important points. We need:

1. A health care practitioner who cares for us, who can see the pattern in our imbalances, who deeply understands the relationship between bodily functions and our mental and emotional natures, and who has enough knowledge and experience in the practice of medicine to prescribe the best and most nontoxic therapies that will help us heal.
2. A hospital or clinic nearby, where surgery or emergency care is provided in a warm, caring, and qualified manner.
3. To know that the care we will need will not bankrupt us, or if it costs us a lot of money, there is assistance in our community to help us get going again.

There is an increasing disparity between these needs and the increasing financial and intellectual rigidity in medicine. This generates much unnecessary conflict. The cornerstone of medicine is the intimate and trusting encounter of patient and practitioner. Many factors today disrupt this sacred encounter. Among these are arrogance, greed, desire to control, and rigidity of thinking. These descriptions apply equally to the medical profession and corporate health care. The next chapter explores a way through these dilemmas.

Remember, your health is your number one asset. We must work now to change our system so it supports this asset in everyone, and thereby lifts the productivity and spirit of all Americans.

Chapter 3

THE FUTURE OF HEALTH CARE

NOW THAT WE have looked at and understood the deficiencies of our current health care system, let us explore what it will require to bring it back into balance. There are no one-shot solutions. We must fundamentally and simultaneously change both the structure and the economics of health care. Doing one without the other will not succeed. To achieve effective and affordable health care, we must establish comprehensive medicine as the primary form of medicine, and we must create Healthy Medicine Associations as economic structures for the new medicine.

Unless our current medical model is fundamentally changed to one of comprehensive medicine, affordable health care will be impossible, regardless of the manipulation of figures, finances, and accounting. Without that change, it will just be about moving numbers around. Without changing the structures and the agreements on responsibilities, all the parties will be able to stay hidden behind a facade that hides real motives and the relationships will stay adversarial.

To make these necessary changes, we must adopt the Seven Core Principles of Healthy Medicine:

1. The primary purpose of medicine is healing. The human being is at the heart of health care economics.
2. Comprehensive medicine as the primary form of medicine; it is the only form that can deliver effective and affordable health care.

3   Freedom for each individual to choose his or her primary care practitioner. The options include M.D.s, D.O.s, N.D.s, D.C.s, L.A.c.s, and other certified practitioners.

4.   Mutual responsibility for both patient and practitioner. Freedom is always accompanied by responsibility. This includes personal responsibility for lifestyle changes, and corporate responsibility to make healthy products and provide healthy services. Healthy economic life is the shared responsibility of every person.

5.   Healthy Medicine Associations that include patients, practitioners, and suppliers in collaborative economic and working relationships. Decentralized, localized care, financed locally and regionally. Staffed by collaborative teams of interdisciplinary practitioners trained in integrative care. These associations are characterized by accountability and transparency of finances. This generates trust, competence, and professional responsibility.

6.   Sustainable Wellness Programs. These would exist in all locales and undertake evaluations not only of people's blood pressure and other measures of health as it is now, but also of homes, environments, products, and workplaces to determine the deeper illness-generating causes such as mold, chemical toxins, heavy metal toxins, dental toxins, and pernicious electromagnetic effects.

7.   Gradual replacement of boards of licensure with certification examinations that demonstrate proficiency in a field of training.

These seven principles can guide us to the correct way to reorganize our economics, so that the economics serve the healing, rather than the reverse. To paraphrase the Bible, the law was made for people, not people for the law.

We can prevent health care costs from spiraling by putting into place a comprehensive medicine model with new economic agreements and collaborations, according to these seven principles.

          The Need   ⟶   Healthy Medicine

          The Model   ⟶   Comprehensive Medicine

Why is replacing allopathic medicine with comprehensive medicine so important? Because it changes what is called the "field." What does this mean? It might bring to mind "the playing field." In addition, physics has used this term for many years. A field is demonstrated when we put iron filings around a magnet and the filings are drawn to that magnet. Auras are another example of fields. Kirlian photography from Russia is able to photograph fields of electron movement around a physical object. The heat from a fire is a field we can feel. When the fire is out, we no longer feel this field of warmth.

Medicine's field in this sense of the word "field" is cold, contracted, and controlled, which reinforces fear in most of us. With comprehensive medicine in place and the financial structure changing, the field can open and let in more warmth. This warmth is the renewed relationship of patient and health care practitioner, with movement toward healing rather than suppression. We may say that the field is open for healing.

The field is kept open by a deep commitment to the core principles of healthy medicine, especially the principles of freedom and responsibility. The field is open when we can relax internally, knowing that there is enough of what we deeply need in life—love, health care, and money, to give three examples—and that healing ourselves will not bankrupt us.

The model for health care is currently excessively based on the function of a machine. This means that medicine treats the body as a machine, removing defective parts and, with drugs, changing defects in the machine's functioning. It also means that, economically, health care functions like a machine.

What steps can we take now?

1. Put the comprehensive medicine model at the core of primary medicine.
2. Reallocate funds that are going toward the type of expensive cardiovascular, cancer, and end-of-life services discussed in the

previous chapter. This means our health care finances must decrease dependency on drugs, surgery, and hospital testing.

3.   Make fundamental changes in health insurance, which is the heart of the economics of health care.

Hold Town Meetings

It is time to have meetings about these important issues. The Emerson Center for Healthy Medicine, Inc., a nonprofit organization based in Prescott, Arizona, and with which I am associated, is sponsoring a series of town meetings throughout the country, so that we may engage in a meaningful dialogue about health care. (See the calendar and address on the web site at www.healthymedicine.org.) The purpose of these meetings is:

1.   To bring all that is hidden to the surface.
2.   To ask questions about how these issues are to be dealt with. In this, we must be willing to be silent, to wait for answers. Today, because we are so conditioned to quick fixes, we ask questions and then want quick solutions. These are not possible in resolving the economic dilemmas of our health care or in healing our chronic illnesses.
3.   To develop real solutions to these problems. For this, we must be aware of the underlying causes of the problems and know that solving them will require change, often big changes, in our lives.

Areas of Change

Change will need to occur in individual lifestyles, the prevailing medical model, corporate medicine, and government.

CHANGES IN INDIVIDUAL LIFESTYLES

We will not have effective, affordable, and fair health care unless enough people and businesses commit to making fundamental changes at home and at work. This means that we take account of lifestyle habits that contribute to the development of illness, and begin to move toward changing these habits. This is the core of individual responsibility. It is what Ralph Waldo Emerson spoke about in his essay, "Self-Reliance." We cannot demand that institutions—business, health care, or government—pay for the consequences of our imbalanced lifestyles. Part 3 of my book *Healthy Medicine* provides the reader with details and depth of understanding in how to make these necessary changes, changes that will help us feel better about ourselves.

CHANGES IN THE ATTITUDES OF RETIREES

People might have to work longer before retirement and their work might be for less income than they are used to under our current model. In the future, it might also be necessary for families or people to live together under one roof, have community meals, and so forth. We have become so entrained into thinking of retirement as one or two people having the life of comfort after sweating at work all those years. Unfortunately, too many of us put off until the future the joys of daily life. Lifestyle changes might also involve doing a home vegetable garden, becoming more self-sufficient, or being involved in a community food garden.

It is unclear whether retirees are willing to make such changes. The level of denial and wanting to live the same illness-generating lifestyles is very strong today. This crisis is compelling all retirees, however, to look seriously at how they spend money. Specifically, how much do you spend on gambling? On eating unhealthy foods? On drug costs? On real estate speculation?

If retirees demand to have things continue as they have been, then everyone will lose. Cities will fall apart out of financial losses. Retirees will have worse health, partially because of their held anger and resentment about how things turned out, and partially because they still feel isolated and fearful of the costs and consequences of illness.

Bottom line, either we change now or circumstances are going to force us to change.

> "Catharsis can be born of consciousness. It does not have to hit the wall of catastrophe." —Christopher Budd, *Rare Albion* (available through www.steinerbooks.org)

Change of Medical Model

The model for paying health care benefits needs to change from allopathic medicine to comprehensive medicine. For this to happen, it is imperative that organizations that represent public employee retirees move to demand that their insurance policies include comprehensive medicine and that Medicare do the same. Organizations need to break free of the medical hypnotism of today and demand that people have the option of products and therapies from comprehensive practitioners covered in their health care policies.

Corporate Medicine Changes

In comprehensive medicine, the health care corporation purchases and invests in capital expenditures in a custodial spirit, rather than in one of ownership. The ownership of equipment used for health diagnosis and treatment is seen as a social responsibility rather than an individual aggrandizement, as it is under our current model.

All involved in health care need to be more aware of the motives and effects of our economic actions on the community and the environment. One must ask, directly, whether thought is given in corporate medicine boardrooms to the effect of rising health care costs that cities allocate for retirees and the effects of this on the very fabric of city life and work.

Two crucial changes that must happen in corporate medicine are:

- Managers must adopt financial transparency as the norm. The mandate for this must come from the top, or managers, for fear of losing their jobs, will continue in the old ways.
- Stockholders must become active participants, in the sense that they are cognizant of the full ramifications, either constructive or destructive, of corporate activities on the health, environment, and economics of the country.

We need to now ask how we can develop a form of capitalism that operates differently: a form that takes into account the hidden costs of pollution, disease, and faulty economics that our current system has been perpetrating; a form that values human labor and creativity. This will take systemic reevaluation by corporate managers and by "regular people" all over the country who are stockholders.

GOVERNMENT CHANGES

The first change that could have a huge impact is for retirees who are eligible for Medicare to demand collectively that the system pay for or reimburse comprehensive medicine practitioners. This means that retired Medicare patients need to shift their focus from demanding to be taken care of, by whatever specialists are available, and instead participate as contributing elders in associations. Specifically, this requires a commitment to break dependence gradually on pharmaceutical drugs, surgeries, and specialty tests. These comprise an enormous expense in health care, and most elderly people are not really served by this arrangement.

The New Health Care System

The main differences in a health care system based on comprehensive medicine compared to our current system will be effectiveness and affordability.

An effective health care system is one that:

* Helps people heal chronic illness.
* Trains practitioners to practice comprehensive medicine.
* Encourages responsibility and self-autonomy.
* Engenders trust.

Healing chronic illness means more than the physical presence of the disease no longer being present. It also means that the person has healed something deeper inside, a wound often from early in life, which opened the door to this chronic illness. Ultimately, this must be our focus. This must be our gift to each other. This unbinds the entanglements in our souls and gives our spirits the chance to reach their full potential of expression in this life, so that others may also be touched by this warmth. Without doing this, we continue to suffer. We must embrace the full depth of the term "healing chronic illness."

Affordability means that comprehensive medicine programs are in place in businesses, insurance programs, and government programs as the first line of health care evaluations and treatments, barring an emergency.

What will be the economic impact of these changes?

* Hospitals and outpatient facilities will see decreased revenue from what they have come to depend on as main revenue sources: cardiovascular procedures and cancer therapies. There will be increased revenue from enhanced comprehensive medicine practices in local hospitals and clinics, and these revenues will remain local, thus supporting local economies.

- Employment in such areas will decrease. Communities can commit, however, to retraining people for the needed work in the hospital of the future.
- Pharmaceutical companies, health insurance companies, and other health industry portfolios will decrease in value, which will affect stock portfolios. Investors will have to readdress the value of stock portfolios, if they choose to continue to invest in pharmaceuticals.

Let's look at what a comprehensive medical model offers economically and in terms of care in comparison to what we get under the current system.

Health Care Now: Restricted Options

When a person does not feel well, he or she goes to the doctor. This is most often the doctor that is on the patient's insurance plan, or a doctor for whose visit the patient can get reimbursed. Except for a few states, this severely restricts the patient's options to the narrow confines of allopathic medicine with its artificially high prices. This means no naturopaths, homeopaths, or acupuncturists—the type of practitioners who treat the causes of illness and not just the symptoms.

Remember, reader, that this situation exists not because of bad insurance companies and bad doctors, but because we have collectively created and agreed on this system. The system would not exist as it is unless most people believed that getting rid of symptoms is the goal of medicine, and that their lifestyles and habits have nothing to do with their illness. This is the current illusion. We can change this anytime we want, by changing our own lifestyles first, and then by changing our economic relationships from excessive competition to collaboration and association. Currently, we drop our driven and destructive economic competitiveness only during crises, such as the aftermath of Hurricane Katrina. It is time to build this behavior into our daily economic lives. This is explained in the pages that follow.

At the doctor visit, a plan is developed for diagnostic evaluation and treatment. Again, this must be approved by insurance plans or the patient's pocketbook is responsible. And again, these procedures and treatments are virtually all allopathic: X-rays, CT scans, lab tests, pharmaceutical drugs. This approach is not looking for deeper causes, but rather is looking for treatments to make symptoms go away. That way, the patient is happy and the doctor gets paid. I called this setup "mutual denial."

As I've noted, these allopathic measures are sometimes needed, an over-reliance on them dooms any attempt to change the finances of health care so it is more affordable to everyone. This fact cannot be overemphasized. Some specific monetary issues to keep in mind are that the average corporate insurance plan for an individual costs $4,500 per year and for a family of four it costs $14,000 per year. To compute the costs of health care for people under such plans, it is necessary to determine what is and isn't covered and what their deductible is.

In comprehensive medicine, the view is much broader and deeper than it is in conventional medicine. The practitioner is looking for the deeper causes of any illness—and there are always more than one—as well as disturbances in organ and tissue function that are at the root of most diseases. Practitioners spend considerably more time talking with and listening to patients. Patients like this, which is why conventional medical schools are emphasizing this now also.

We must take note here, again, that most people have spent a lifetime ignoring their illness-generating habits. So it may take time and energy to find the deeper causes and address them. This needs a new economic arrangement.

There are often more laboratory and other tests in comprehensive medicine than in conventional medicine. In addition to standard lab tests, there may be such testing as the following:

- Hair mineral analysis to evaluate for general metabolic function, nutritional deficiencies, and heavy metal toxicity.
- Comprehensive blood tests, looking for subtle irregularities.
- Nutritional evaluations, far more specific than those of conventional medicine.
- Thermography, a safe and effective way to evaluate for the presence of early breast cancer.
- Urine tests for organic acids, indicating toxic exposures and effect on cellular chemistry.
- Plasma amino acids, to evaluate protein needs.
- Office urine and saliva testing, to determine biochemical disturbances.

After such testing, treatment programs are then developed by the practitioner, and proposed to the patient. These are highly individualized programs that require much more patient participation than just taking pills. (Comprehensive medicine testing and treatments are discussed in depth in *Healthy Medicine,* and will not be discussed further here.)

Comprehensive medicine tests need to be made a priority in most illnesses, long before expensive CT scans, MRIs, and PET scans are ordered. This scenario will save us much money, and ensure that we will be addressing the causes of illness and not just treating the physical changes that result from illness.

Relying on these tests will also mean that the private companies that have been starting up everywhere to offer MRIs and private surgical centers will be much less needed. This will, of course, hurt the investors in these enterprises, and there are many interests in this country that do not want this to happen. These investors include not just large doctor groups, but also many readers with mutual funds. Each of us will have to address the impact of these changes. As one of the signers of the Declaration of Independence said, we must all hang together or we shall certainly all hang separately. This applies just as much in this time of significant change, even though the threat to each of us is not being physically hung but rather being hung economically and medically.

Most, if not all, comprehensive medicine tests and the treatments to correct the imbalances, depending on the license of the practitioner, are not covered by private insurance, Medicare, nor Medicaid. In the instances they are, the decisions are made based on rigid economic formulas that do not permit individual practitioners to do what they do best: support real healing in patients. Changing this in a deep and far-reaching way is the necessity if our health care is to become more effective and more affordable. It will be necessary for individuals and businesses to demand that this care be covered by insurance policies. But this is only the first step.

In addition, the entire way that decisions are made by insurance regulators and government health care regulators will have to change. At the present time, in private health insurance companies, a person on a phone somewhere else in the country from where you see the doctor makes an arbitrary decision about whether your insurance covers a test or treatment. This arbitrariness is based on decisions made higher up in the insurance company, by managers and administrators whose jobs depend on keeping investors happy by keeping returns high.

In comprehensive medicine, as we will see in subsequent pages, decision-making will be quite different. Without the driving controlling forces of distant market economics behind research institutions, clinics, and hospitals, practitioners will make decisions that are based on comprehensive medicine practices (see my book *Healthy Medicine*), and will choose effective and affordable therapies from a much wider range of options that include, but are not restricted to, current allopathic medicine.

A THIRD WAY, A MIDDLE PATH

The breakdown in the twin pillars of health care—health care financing and quality health care—is now extending into the lives of millions of Americans. It is unfortunate this is happening. The good that can come of this, however, is that the dirty laundry is now more out in the open.

The two current polarities we are facing in health care in 2006 are private health insurance, either employee-based on individual, and government-financed insurance. To be sure, employer-based health insurance is also government based in part, not directly, but through tax subsidies.

The first of these, private health insurance, has proven to be a patchwork of increasingly unmanageable, complex, restrictive, and expensive way of financing health care. As discussed, this form of insurance only exists today because of massive hidden government subsidies. These hidden subsidies prop up private employer-based health insurance to the tune of $190 billion per year. Without it, there would be no private employer health insurance. It is a subsidy for thousands of families, a tax break. In other words, the benefits are not taxed, yet wages are taxed. This hidden federal subsidy saves the typical family of four whose income is in the $75,000 to $100,000 range about $4,000 per year.

In other words, while local governments are financially stressed by Medicaid and promises for health benefits to retirees, and Medicare is stressed by an increasingly aging population, those families who make $100,000 receive a federal tax subsidy to pay for health insurance through employer-based corporate insurance.

But do these families really benefit from this $4,000 saved? Premiums rise, deductibles rise, uncovered services rise, insurance companies arbitrarily decide what and what not to cover and make it more difficult for doctors to accept such insurance, and increasingly debilitating illnesses bankrupt more and more families who thought they were covered.

Increasingly, many of these families with incomes of greater than $100,000 per year are actually in a cash-flow crunch, having invested most savings in precarious real estate, and having virtually nothing for unexpected events like job loss or incapacitating illness, let alone for retirement.

The alternative to private health insurance, an alternative suggested by a growing number of people, is a government single-payer plan. This has not made much headway in part because corporation-driven deceitfulness has misled most Americans into thinking that government spending is the root of all evil. Even though without such spending there would be no good roads, no trash pickups, no airport protection, no public libraries, and a lack of many other essential services. The Harry and Louise advertisements run by the health insurance industry in the early 1990s, when the Clinton administration attempted to increase the federal role in health care, is a clear example of this deceitfulness.

It highlights the fundamental struggle in the psyche of America: Who best should manage land and services? Most Americans at this time would unequivocally say that the private sector should. But the private sector today is not what most people still perceive as the private sector. The private sector today is greed run amuck. This seriously compromises health care for millions of Americans.

At the same time, there is very little independent, dispassionate government that speaks for the common man and woman. Most governmental intrusions into the private lives of Americans today, especially at the federal level, are driven by hidden corporate forces. Consistently, all three branches of the federal government now make the rule of law stand for and support the excesses of predator-like and greed-driven competitive, market share economics. This pervades health care as it pervades most aspects of our lives. This way of doing things does not work in health care if our goal is to improve the health and well-being of our people.

Fortunately, there is a third way, neither corporate nor governmental. Our health care problems are systemic. They go beyond the paradigm of business and labor, private and public. The third way requires us to form new associations and a new paradigm. The third way is the formation of what I call Healthy Medicine Associations. The purpose of these associations is to support healing in all participants, and permit the health care practitioners to do the work in which they are skilled and which they love.

Healthy Medicine Associations would be local community-based organizations that are also connected and interrelated with such organizations all over the country. The formation of these associations is unlike other forms of business: these entities are associative, or collaborative. What this means is that the structure of these organizations derives from the working together of three sectors that are today competitive and often adversarial. These three sectors are:

1. Consumers, or patients and their families.
2. Providers, or health care practitioners.
3. Suppliers, or hospitals, hospital supply companies, pharmaceutical companies, and nutritional supplement companies.

The concept of medical associations is not original to me. It derives from the movement to develop what is called a civil society. Associations in this context are organizations devoted to the development of sustainable culture, and are outside of, but not in opposition to, both traditional government and modern business enterprises. The central idea here is that health care's proper place is not in the economic realm of life, driven by market forces that artificially drive up costs, nor is it in the government realm, where excessive laws and regulations constrict freedom of care. The true home of health care is in the cultural realm, along with education, spirituality, religion, and the creative arts. The reader can discover more on associations and civil society by entering these words into an internet search engine.

How would Healthy Medicine Associations work?

Patients and their families, health care practitioners, and suppliers meet and decide what is fair. This issue of fairness is rarely talked about in our present system, but it is a centerpiece of Healthy Medicine Associations. Prices need to be fair and affordable to all parties. They are not now, because the market in health care today has many hidden elements that permit corporate greed to flourish and government to increase control. These meetings, which form the basis of Healthy Medicine Associations, can start to take place in business meeting rooms, community meeting rooms, religious institutions, and local government buildings.

The creation of Healthy Medicine Associations represents a fundamental shift in health care from a top-down system of authoritarian control by various interest groups and governmental agencies aligned with them, which often operate today in callous ways, into a bottom-up health care system. The current big players would become the middlemen, the suppliers, not the controllers. This fundamental shift is much needed. If the Healthy Medicine Association decided that the local hospital needed to be stocked with herbs and supplements as well as drugs, then this would happen. In addition, the economic arrangements, including all contracts, would be transparent at all times, available for anyone to review, and would be characterized by complete accountability.

This is not socialism or communism. It actually is capitalism functioning in a healthy way, with many private businesses providing goods and services, and with many individual and group practices composed of practitioners who would still have to practice within the guidelines of certification parameters. The difference is that people involved in the associations—patients and their families, practitioners, and suppliers—would decide these parameters. And they would decide how funds are to be collected and spent on health care.

The basic tenets of a Healthy Medicine Association need to be:

1. It is not formed by health care practitioners, but rather by a partnership of patients and practitioners. Practitioners will not initiate this movement; the movement toward forming such an association needs to come from the public. In this way, from the beginning, practitioners and patients, along with suppliers, are partners.

2. There is transparency of finances. This means that the agreements formed and signed for such an association, and the financial management and accounting books of the association, are open for any to see and review. This also means, in practical terms, that the full expenses of an association clinic are revealed in the agreements, so that all who participate can understand the financial structure of the association and the reasons for the expenses.

3. It will be clear that, for their membership fee, members receive much more in professional services in a year than the same amount would purchase in single visits. The services covered by the membership fee include initial and a certain number of follow-up visits with the doctor and other therapists, and diagnostic testing done in the office. Laboratory testing and X-rays might also be included, as well as homeopathic remedies and supplements from the pharmacy. There would need to be provisions for the use of more expensive allopathic testing and treatments when necessary. This is currently what we call "catastrophic care protection." But if we incorporate this comprehensive medicine model and move to an associative model, the costs of catastrophic protection will drop significantly, with much lower deductibles. The costs will drop because the hospitals where people go for such care will not be beholden to big corporate interests. In addition, members could have unlimited access to therapies that do not require the practitioner to be present, such as microcurrent or sauna therapies. The services covered could vary from one association to another, but are clearly defined for patients. There will also be payment options for all members.

4. There is an agreement between patients, families, health care practitioners, and suppliers as to what the responsibilities of all parties are. Patients have such responsibilities as attending classes in health education and making commitments to lifestyle changes, so that health care costs can be lowered. The practitioners are responsible for delivering quality patient care that complies with current licensing and certification requirements.

The responsibilities of suppliers are to provide quality products, verified by independent testing. This is already occurring in the nutritional supplement industry with Good Manufacturing Practices (GMP). Suppliers are also responsible for maintaining transparent financial and accounting practices. The current resistance of most insurance companies and hospitals to disclosing the real costs of services and products they provide must dissolve. So much good will come to all of us when there is no longer the need, personally and in business and government, to keep things hidden.

The thinking behind the Healthy Medicine Association model is that to deliver the best possible care to each person, it is best if the medical staff is not spending time balancing books. They need to focus on serving the needs of their patients and remove themselves from the business of medicine. That business needs to be done by association members who understand that arena.

It is important to note here that in locally based health associations, with networks of practitioners and patients collaborating in unified endeavors, there must be a freedom of choice for all practitioners to practice and see patients in the space that each deems best. We see this today in the small, quiet, and sacred spaces in which many acupuncturists, body workers, and herbalists work with their patients. It is imperative to maintain this integrity.

Too often we think of health care in terms of hospitals and large clinics. There is still a need for these, of course. But we must create small sacred spaces within these large buildings, so that the warmth and intimacy that characterize the true healing encounter can be maintained and nurtured, and not be overwhelmed as it is too often today by the business of health care. This big business, in the throes of greed-driven market forces, is often devoid of spirit.

The Economics of Healthy Medicine Associations

For this model to work, everyone involved needs to make changes. Many people would be required to change their lifestyle toward healthier products and habits, as part of their responsibility as a member of a Healthy Medicine Association, as a price for having freedom of choice of practitioner. The current capacity on the part of many people to demand any and all testing, however expensive, and have some other agency pay for it, would be eliminated.

This is not control, nor is it rationing. It is having healthy boundaries to our wants and desires. It is thinking of more than ourselves, thinking of how our economic lives affect the economic lives of others. This is healthy. The reason that it would not be rationing is that there would not be a scarcity of funds for comprehensive medicine care. The savings from the changes in the medical system could be transferred to the associations. For example, huge savings would result from: 1) tremendously lower bureaucratic expenses of hundreds of private insurance companies; 2) the elimination of the federal tax subsidy for employer-based health insurance; and 3) significant reduction in the number of expensive procedures and treatments, such as stents, bypass grafts, and new-generation cancer drugs. All of this points to having funds available for such associations that we do not think about today. We could have teams of health care thinkers and planners, independent of corporate and government employment, work with economists to develop a new economic model for a comprehensive medical model.

There would be no insurance companies deciding on care based on rigid and arbitrary rules, with the main agenda of providing big profits to stockholders. The members of these Healthy Medicine Associations would be the stockholders and distributors of funds for health care, to member patients, health care practitioners, and providers (hospitals, pharmaceuticals, medical supply companies).

There would, of course, be many businesses and corporations in health care, but these would no longer control the purse strings. Such companies, to stay in business, would have to make products and provide services that members of associations want. And these members would be motivated to good health by contracting with companies that enable them to keep prices fair and reasonable.

Health care practitioners in the Healthy Medicine Associations would be paid a fair price for services. Payment would have flexibility and variability depending on participants and locality. But the principle of freedom of choice of practitioner would be sacrosanct.

For these changes to take place, the consumer of health care must insist on prices such that people can afford to sell and buy what they mutually need. Today, the "normal" way of seeking health care is to seek the lowest-priced care, so that the consumer can get more for his or her money. But the same consumer is also a producer. This way of thinking, of always looking for the lowest-priced care, means that at the same time the consumer must work longer hours and get lower prices for what he or she offers.

In this all-too-common scenario, we are each like a rat on a turning wheel, trying to find the lowest prices for what we must purchase, yet making less income because others are seeking lower prices from us. This does not work. No one feels valued, and everyone is competing with everyone else, so sees everyone else as a threat. In health care, it means that people will try to find care that is cheapest but not necessarily the best. So we will seek a short visit with a doctor and buy a couple of supplements, instead of doing the deeper work of healing, which takes longer and requires more money.

For health care to become more affordable and effective, it not only needs to be comprehensive, that is, it utilizes both what today is called alternative medicine and conventional medical modalities when needed. In addition, the stigma of money needs to be removed from the short-term decision-making. This enables patients to come to offices and be open and receptive for healing, and enables practitioners to administer tests and treatments necessary for the patient. With the increase in integrative and energy medicine diagnostic and therapeutic modalities, much can now be done in-house, in clinic offices, and be included under the care plan. Health care used to be this way, until pharmaceutical- and surgery-driven medicine drove up prices so much as to make basic care unaffordable to many. A Healthy Medicine Association works to restore the balance of effective and affordable care.

Delivering the best care sometimes takes the practitioner only 15 minutes with a patient, whereas at other times the practitioner knows that it may take one to two hours. Practitioners need to be free to prescribe according to these perceptions. The only way this can occur is if the stigma of paying for visits by the length of time per visit is removed.

Most comprehensive medicine practitioners are aware of the uniqueness of each individual and of the need not to fall into the trap of treating the disease instead of addressing the unique situation of each patient. The latter approach requires time and effort. It is vital that this time and effort not have the Sword of Damocles, the Clock, hanging over the two people—practitioner and patient—who are engaged in a healing journey.

The guiding economic principles in Healthy Medicine Associations include:

1. Making prices affordable for all parties.
2. Investing only where there is a need for investment; discontinuing speculative investment.
3. Engendering realistic expectations, not demands and excessive wants. This is setting healthy boundaries and means changing our economic life in health care from self-centeredness to being aware of others and how our decisions and actions affect them and affect the environment.
4. Integrating heartfelt principles into the financing of health care.

Under this model, wasteful private health insurance and excessive governmental regulation of health care would be gone. What we will need then is some form of universal coverage that includes both crisis protection, called catastrophic insurance, and personal health care insurance, through the Healthy Medicine Associations I propose.

In the necessary transition from private health insurance and government-financed health care to health associations, members of a health association could have several financial options. If they already have health insurance, then they could raise their deductible and invest the money saved in joining the association. This would mean saving, for example, $1,500 per person in order to do so. In the event of a catastrophic problem, the person or family would be responsible for more of the costs of a hospital or surgeon than before because their deductible is higher. But by investing in a membership in a health association that is based on comprehensive medicine, many people will decrease their need for expensive care.

Individuals who do not have health insurance would be required to pay membership fees. Membership fees could be paid monthly, quarterly, or all at once, with a sliding fee scale for low-income people.

What If?

One of my mentors asks participants in his seminars to train practitioners in comprehensive medicine practices to consider the following questions. I offer them for your consideration:

What if you knew you were insured, meaning protected from the financial ravages of illness and supported in doing the work of healing?

What if you knew you could go to the health care practitioner of your choice?

What would you be willing to do in order to have this reality in your life?

What would you be willing to change in your daily life, relationships, and habits?

Would you be willing to change your current insurance care deductible to a higher amount in order to become a member of a health care association that, by you engaging actively in its health-promoting activities, would decrease your risk of becoming ill enough to have to use the hospital and expensive laboratory testing?

Are you willing to take this risk, for the betterment of your own health, that of your loved ones, and that of everyone in this society?

Can you embrace this enlarged egoism?

In summary, the present way of practicing health care in this country cannot survive. We need to have something constructive in place as the current allopathic medical paradigm collapses. *Beyond the Medical Meltdown* is intended to support this process. The idea here is to go beyond the ineffective and unaffordable medicine of our present model, and even the relatively new integrative clinic model, to create a new way of practicing, one that brings together consumers (patients), producers (practitioners), and intermediary suppliers in an associative way. This approach enables the delivery of quality care and we all benefit. (Remember, all practitioners and all suppliers are also patients at one time or another.)

By establishing these associations, we can begin to extricate the holy practice of medicine from the entanglements of greed-driven economic engines that are now called normal, and return this holy art of healing to its proper domain: that of supporting each individual in transforming life through the healing of illness, and support the delivery of this care with healthy, commonsense economics.

When this movement toward health care associations becomes more of a reality, then the field of health care will attract more people for whom health care is a calling, a field in which to express one's deeper purpose rather than only being a way to make a living.

It must be emphasized again that the comprehensive medicine model goes far beyond, though includes, what most people understand as today's alternative medicine: diet, nutritional supplements, chiropractic, and acupuncture. As Dr. David Eisenberg's studies at Harvard have shown, this is where the great majority of funds have gone in alternative medicine in the first five years of the twenty-first century.

Comprehensive medicine, in order to deliver effective care, must include:

- Homeopathic medicine: Though slandered by modern medicine as being merely placebo, homeopathy has a rich tradition and written history of thousands of cases of successful healing, in chronic illness and in acute pandemics like the flu pandemic of 1918.
- Herbal medicine: The public will have to understand that the headline stories that appear in the media today about the alleged harms of certain herbal medicines pale to insignificance when compared with the number of people who die each year from pharmaceuticals, as reported in the *Journal of the American Medical Association.*
- Holistic dentistry: This comprehensive dental care recognizes that mercury amalgam fillings, root canals, bite problems, hidden bone infections, and other areas of modern dentistry that are ignored by most dentists and doctors are key elements in the generation of chronic illness. Today, most dentistry, like conventional medicine, focuses on where the money is (orthodontics, whitening of teeth, and periodontal surgeries) and ignores the illness-generating consequences of its procedures and the industry persecution of holistic dentists.

There are many permutations and pathways that can take us from where we are now to where we need to be, including any number of the following:

- University integrative medicine programs develop a backing.
- One or more major corporate self-insurers move toward a comprehensive medicine model of care.
- Local governments begin to set up associative economic arrangements, and invite meetings of patients, providers, and

suppliers of health care to dialogue. Local funds then begin to be allocated to such organizations.

- State-financed Medicaid programs change such that they include alternative practitioners in comprehensive programs and ask all participants to be part of associations based on the core principles of healthy medicine.
- Large and midsized employers start to see the wisdom in such arrangements. They realize that the comprehensive medicine model will lower their health care costs and assure that they will have happier and more productive employees. These companies step in to create associative organizations within their businesses, which are then part of networks of collaborative associations between businesses, bringing together employees and their families; these are new provider networks based on the model of comprehensive medicine. After dialogues and number-crunching, these businesses then negotiate with local hospitals for services and demand that their insurance carriers include comprehensive medicine with freedom of choice of primary practitioner.
- Small business owners, who are especially vulnerable to rising health care costs because, unlike large corporations, they cannot absorb the costs of even one employee having large medical bills for a serious illness, demand the change to comprehensive medicine as the predominant model of health care, with conventional medicine as secondary medicine, utilized when a life-threatening emergency or need for surgery arises or when other forms of healing fail. Small businesses change their economic perspective from being a victim of insurance/hospital/ pharmaceutical control and distant decision-making to being actively involved with forming new health care arrangements with employees and health care providers.

CONCLUSION

IT IS THE time for us to make bold moves, like the ones suggested in these pages. It is time for us to work toward fundamentally altering the way we practice medicine and how we finance it. For the ideas outlined in this book to become a reality, we must move toward:

- Making comprehensive medicine the primary medicine.
- Assuring that all hospitals fully practice comprehensive medicine.
- Creating Healthy Medicine Associations, with membership fees, mutual agreements, and transparent accounting finances
- Transferring funds away from unnecessary cardiovascular and cancer therapies.
- Financing associations offering freedom of choice in health care practitioners.
- Eliminating all tax breaks for families for health insurance, and replacing them with affordable and effective association care.
- Opening comprehensive medical centers and staffing them with people well trained in integrative and energy medicine.
- Establishing a network of comprehensive medicine practitioners.
- Beginning services to inspect homes for causes of illness.
- Lifting the veil on our incorrect assumptions that: modern medicine helps people heal, most people are healthy, the cause of most illness is genetic and/or biochemical and can be fixed at that level, and getting rid of symptoms equals better health.

Let's look for a moment at the last item on this list. The reality is that modern medicine does not focus on healing, regardless of the words that advertisements use. Modern medicine is focused on the quick fix that makes uncomfortable symptoms disappear with drugs or surgery, and on making as much profit as possible while keeping people under control and providing as little services in as quick a time as possible. There is little healing in such a system.

The second reality is that most people today are ill. This does not necessarily mean physical organic pathological illness such as cancer or heart disease. It means that most of us have functional imbalances in our biochemistry, physiology, and psyches, which are the soil in which pathological illnesses develop. Most people are toxic with chemicals, heavy metals, and biological organisms, as well as being deficient in many essential nutrients. This is disease in the process of becoming.

The third reality is that the cause of most illness is not genetic or biochemical, but the causes just listed. Genetic changes and biochemical imbalances are the results of these factors. The reason for the genetic and biochemical focus in medicine is that this is where the greatest profit can be made in pharmaceuticals, hospital technologies, and genetic research.

The fourth reality is that getting rid of symptoms might make us feel more comfortable with less pain, but it does not give us better health. It takes time, energy, and, yes, money to heal. Achieving better health means making deep commitments to change the way we do things.

The future of medicine, if it is to be effective and affordable, requires us to recognize and act on the recognition that health care is a healing journey. To undertake and do our best with this journey, we need help. This means collaborating with others, including professionals, who can help us in our efforts to heal. Currently, our fear- and scarcity-based health care system does not support us in these ways. To change that, we must liberate health care from its economic tyranny and establish new forms of collaboration. We need to set up a quite different process, so that a sacred space is created in which both patient and practitioner can do what they need to do, which is to focus on healing.

This book has discussed how to change the economics of health care. Doing this is not a quick fix. It requires us to consider what is involved, to be willing to look at situations, and hold ourselves in check from immediately drawing clever conclusions. It means that we must be honest about motives, our own and those of pharmaceutical companies, hospitals, and insurance companies. It means we must deeply reevaluate how we look at health care.

It is the responsibility of each of us to do our best in self-regulating our lifestyles and becoming autonomous. At the same time, it is also our responsibility to recognize how our thoughts, words, and actions have an impact on others. More specifically, if we continue to think that our health care economy is healthy and only needs tweaking, we are in serious denial. We are currently in the midst of an epidemic of suppression on all levels. We suppress our deepest emotions and feelings when revealing them would threaten our comfortable lifestyles of denial; we suppress our discomfort at seeing the suffering of others; we suppress our creative capacities under a cultural blanket of conformity and fear. This suppression has become so pervasive as to appear normal. We must find the will to work together to emerge from this denial and suppression into fuller, more creative lives.

Earlier in this book, I mentioned Wendell Berry's comments on how to bring about fundamental, healthy social change. He made three points. The first is that there are no piecemeal changes. This is true in health care and in our individual lives. Humans are complex and mysterious, and the care of humans requires attention and not piecemeal changes, quick fixes, or mechanistic solutions.

Berry's second point is to walk the talk. If you truly want change, you, the reader, can no longer be misinformed, oblivious, or irresponsible. Walking the talk means that we practice what we preach to others. It means that if we ourselves want help in times of need, then we must be prepared to respond to others in their time of need, as best we can. We cannot in good conscience ask others to live healthy lifestyles and keep health care costs down unless we ourselves do the same.

Berry's final point is to be poor. What does this mean? It means that we must provide inexpensive solutions that are within reach of everyone. This does not mean finding the cheapest vitamin, however. There is a tremendous range in quality of supplements and quality of practitioners. What this statement does mean is that we have at our disposal methods to provide relatively inexpensive care for everyone. But this only happens in a healthy medicine system based on the model of comprehensive medicine, which employs the affordable and effective diagnostic and therapeutic modalities of energy and other natural medicines.

English scientist Rupert Sheldrake has called science "the last unreformed institution in the modern world today," further declaring that, in it, decisions are made by "a small and powerful group of people who are authoritarian, well-funded, entrenched, and see themselves as a priesthood" (*Ode* vol. 3, no. 9, Nov. 2005, pp. 26–31).

This is the condition of modern medicine today, hiding as it does behind the illusion of science. Medical, insurance, and governmental authorities come up with plans and fit people into them. This mechanistic and overly materialistic approach will not work anymore. It is breaking down in health care, education, the arts, prisons, and public utilities and is destroying the environment and making our homes unhealthy with toxic products. Doing things in this way, with life run by authorities that do not selflessly have our best health in mind, leads to further suffering. And not stepping up individually and collaboratively permits people to stay in the same illness-generating lifestyles, full of demands based on unfaced fears and full of expectations based on the past. The institutions that thrive from a growing epidemic of chronic disease depend on our staying this way, frozen in fear and denial.

It is unclear to me whether the will exists to make the necessary changes. There are many people and businesses that benefit from keeping things the way they are. They include:

1. Americans who want to continue eating poor quality food, living unhealthy lifestyles, and demanding that someone else pay for the consequences. These people have the health care system they asked for.

2. Americans who desire to keep their stock portfolios growing, choosing to ignore the fact that this depends on the financial success of insurance companies, pharmaceutical companies, hospital corporations, and the like. Again, these people are helping to keep the health care system as it is.

3. Corporate and union managers, owners, and administrators who clearly benefit from things continuing as they are. This group includes hundreds of thousands of people employed in hospitals, pharmaceutical companies, insurance companies, and government.

4. Physicians who see medicine as merely a way to make a living rather than a call to heal, and who choose to remain in an arrogant and superior state of mind that is condescending to comprehensive medicine.

5. Those contracting the building of hospitals, which are unconscionably being built at a rapid pace, generating huge costs that will be born by individuals and families, and local, state, and federal governments that are already stressed economically in meeting basic needs.

The message that emanates from and is broadcast by modern medicine, in so many ways, is:

> This is the way it is.
> This is the way it is always going to be.
> If you do not like it, get out.

If you accept this model and do not take action, in your own life and with others, to change health care, then most people will be subject to the effects of cutbacks in benefits, deepening personal financial problems due to rising health care costs, worsening of health, and bankrupt cities unable to provide basic services. We need the comprehensive medicine model with the new economic collaborations and agreements discussed in these pages. We need Healthy Medicine.

Rising health care costs and decreasing coverage are bankrupting millions and putting significant financial stress on millions more individual people, small businesses, and local and state governments. This is unnecessary and can be corrected, if we have the courage to take the necessary steps outlined in this book.

Many economists perceive a financially unstable and unpredictable near future for the United States. This is especially true if the housing market cools significantly and interest rates rise. John Wasik, author of *The Kitchen Table Investor,* and a columnist for Bloomberg News (www.bloomberg.com) writes that in 2004, home equity debt was forty percent of the gross domestic product. If the housing market cools and the small gains in personal income continue, many middle-class families will be severely financially stressed, in what Wasik calls a cash-flow poverty. As a result, many people will have less disposable income to spend on health care, and may be thrown on government Medicaid health insurance rolls. This will further stress both the health of individuals and families, and the financial health of businesses and local governments and economies. The health of the economy is deeply connected to the health of people.

We cannot have health care security under the present system of health care. We are living in very insecure times, and the guarantee of security is often a lie of politicians and corporate advertisers. What we need is an economic restructuring of health care on fundamental levels. We cannot separate economy from healing. We have created a speculation-based economy and a health care system that suppresses healing.

In response to the excesses of free market economics in health care, with the resultant financial stress on businesses and individuals, there is a growing interest in some circles for increasing the federal government involvement in health care reform.

One of the main people favoring this direction is Lief Wellington Haase of the Century Foundation in New York City. In *A New Deal for Health,* he proposes universal health coverage, a federally offered private health insurance plan. In this approach, everyone would buy their own private health insurance. But instead of the present way it is being done, with over 1,300 separate private health insurance companies with very confusing policies, there would be a national pool of money that would then be distributed by the federal government to private administrators of health care.

The authors emphasize that this plan is therefore not national health care run by government, but rather a nationally offered private health insurance in which the federal government serves as a collector of funds and as a watchdog, acting in the consumer's best interest to negotiate the largest discount. As Mr. Haase states, "The federal government would sponsor several different insurance options, establish minimum benefit packages, and negotiate with insurers on their price. All plans would offer good coverage of proven benefits.... For every American household, the government will make a contribution to the purchase of a premium for a basic health insurance plan.... Purchasing ... will be mandatory for individuals" (Lief Wellington Haase, "Universal Health Coverage: Coming Sooner Than You Think," *A New Deal for Health,* Century Foundation Press, 2005).

This proposal is a step in the right direction, searching for a middle path between government control of health care and market-driven private insurance inefficiencies. What motivates such proposals is that private market-driven health insurance has left too many individuals and businesses in a financially vulnerable position, and as a result, we now need a structure that will protect people and businesses from these free-market ravages.

But is there any level of government anymore that can serve as an independent and fair collector of funds and as a watchdog acting in the best interests of the consumer? Is there any level of government, especially the federal government, that has not been coopted by corporate health care money influence? Can the federal government be trusted to act as an independent watchdog in the best interests of the consumer?

Until such a government exists, one that acts in the interests of equality and fairness in health care and is free of corporate influence, if this is possible, it is going to be necessary for people and businesses to form independent health associations as described in this book. A growing number of people, including this author, are wondering whether government at either federal or state levels will be solvent in the coming years. With the current levels of national debt and the current federal spending priorities that strongly favor corporate interests, there is reason to suspect that such a federal government would siphon tax funds collected for these proposed national health care pools away from their intended purpose in health care and toward misguided and socially destructive current priorities.

With neither the current market-driven private insurance model nor the government-as-an-independent-representative-of-health-care realistic at this time, it is imperative that we now move toward locally formed health associations. In the troubling times that may be approaching us, we will need to develop new initiatives that are locally based and financed.

If there are positive changes at all levels of government, changes that reestablish trust in government as a representative for equality of rights, then we can at some future time revisit how local health associations can combine and support a more federal universal plan.

To be effective and affordable, this author suggests that health associations be established locally throughout the United States, and that they be based on the Seven Core Principles of Comprehensive Medicine.

We need to establish associations to move us toward sane economics and comprehensive practices in health care. We need people who want to move from a confrontational and fear-based model of health care to a collaborative and trust-based model.

In *The Wizard of Oz,* the Wicked Witch of the West rules through fear and intimidation. Our health care system and our political and economic process, reflects this condition. Dorothy, who represents the Spirit of America, was guided by Goodness to find the Yellow Brick Road, to find the Wizard who would help her get back to Kansas. She found three noble helpers: the straw man (clear thinking), the tin man (heart), and the lion (courage). After the trials, she was able to return to America, her home. Dorothy is that person in all of us who wants to go home, to return to that state of health before things started to get crazy. America has lost its way, in health care and in other areas. Through working together to restore an effective and affordable system of health care, we can help America find its way again.

To borrow from *King, Warrior, Magician, Lover: Rediscovering the Archetypes of the Mature Masculine,* by Robert Moore and Douglas Gillette, we must make four essential transformations on the Yellow Brick Road to a better health care system. We need to change:

- From being intolerant tyrants to beneficent stewards of our own lives and in our corporate boardrooms.
- From fighting to stay in control to surrendering to a commitment to healing.
- From manipulation of information to get ahead and to profit at the expense of others to providing deeper insight into healing.
- From being obsessed with making physical symptoms disappear to exploring artfully the meaning behind these symptoms and being patient in our daily practices.

As Lynne Twist states in *The Soul of Money,* there is no shortage of love, energy, food, and money. And I would add healing. Scarcity is an illusion we have created and which we can correct.

I offer this book in the hope that enough people want to make changes in both their personal and business lives, and want to feel an integrity and consistent morality between these two aspects of themselves. What specifically does this mean we need to be doing? We need to:

1. Learn how to live with uncertainty.
2. Ask questions: Be an informed, free-thinking, active patient and citizen. What products do we consume? What toxins were used in their production? What were the human and ecological costs of production?
3. Question all assumptions. This means such assumptions as:
   - Milk builds strong bones (it does not).
   - Antibiotics cure diseases (they do not).
   - Fluoride prevents tooth decay without harm (it can harm).
   - More drugs mean better health (untrue).
   - There are enough nutrients in our foods (our foods are devitalized of nutrients by decades of soil mismanagement by corporate farming).
4. Have people around us who challenge us to live to our capacity, to be creative, to live more fully in the present, and move our lives from fear to trust.
5. Be grateful—for our troubles and our illnesses for what they can teach us. Give thanks in silence and with patience. Create a bank account of hope.

We cannot know the outcome of our efforts to change and improve health care until we begin to do the work, the practice. Taking the steps outlined in this book involves trust. It reminds me of the young child who, on first standing, unsteady on his feet, does not know at all that he will be able to take the next step. Yet he continues.

We too must now take this step. The old ways will no longer suffice. We must courageously combine head, heart, and will—vision, compassion, and action—to create something new for ourselves. If enough of us take this step of trust to act in collaborative and cooperative ways, we can bring about the fundamental changes proposed in this book.

Appendix A

HEALTHY MEDICINE
AND SUSTAINABILITY

THE COMPREHENSIVE MEDICINE model described in my book *Healthy Medicine: A Guide to the Emergence of Sensible Comprehensive Care* goes hand in hand with healthy economic changes in local agriculture and manufacture. We will need networks of neighborhoods that support healthy medicine, locally grown food, healthy homes and workplaces, and affordable utilities, and meet local needs before exporting products. Indeed, healthy local economy is only sustainable with healthy medicine.

Our economic life is not just numbers, pensions, and retirement. Such a focus generates fear. Our economic life is a living organism, and we need to treat it as such. For it to thrive, the corporations involved in health care need to change to being guided by spiritual principles, and trust that the monies will come if the right principles guide the ship.

The focus in the future will be on renewing local economy. This will require:

- Health care that is comprehensive and economical.
- Foods that are grown locally and organically.
- Products that are nontoxic.
- Houses and other buildings that are healthy and nontoxic.
- Utilities that produce affordable, sustainable, and nontoxic energy and water.

It is sometimes helpful to think about these complex issues in simple ways. For example, the human body must have a healthy circulation in order to function well. This means blood must circulate. If the blood becomes stagnant, or if there are blockages in arteries and veins that prevent its normal flow, then disease develops. This is well known in conventional medicine, and attempts to remedy this are the aim of many drugs and surgeries.

Can we see the economy in the same way we see the human body? In other words, can we ask questions such as: How can we make sure there is a healthy circulation of money for goods and services in a community, and that money is available for lending and investments? A living community has healthy circulation of monies among businesses, education, farming, health care, eldercare, and other enterprises. The point to be made here is that today, with our excessive focus on self-aggrandizement and retirement portfolios, all based on fear of not having enough, we have normalized the hoarding of money. There are billions of dollars in this country that are held tightly in gold, in land, in stocks, and in other forms that inhibit the free flow of monies for healthy communities. This hoarding of money is akin to blood that is stagnant. When this happens in the human body, we see higher blood viscosity and resultant infections and inflammations in the blood vessel walls.

But just as we do in health care—ignore the deeper causes and just give drugs to lower cholesterol or do surgeries that remove blockages—we ignore the deeper causes of our economic difficulties and try for quick fixes that do not exist.

With the comprehensive medicine model of health care in place, along with the economic association model that supports this type of care, the new health care economy will better sustain people in their personal lives and relationships, and in their work and economics. As a result, the creative forces that will be unleashed by these changes will enhance environmental and workplace sustainability.

Appendix B

HEALTH CARE
AND THE SPIRIT OF AMERICA

As THE UNITED States undergoes rapid changes on many levels in the early twenty-first century, let us look at health care through the prism of original American values. The Declaration of Independence begins: "We hold these truths to be self-evident, that all men are created equal, that they are endowed by their Creator with certain unalienable Rights, that among these are Life, Liberty and the pursuit of Happiness."

We may first look at the word "equal." We know this term perhaps best in phrases such as "equal protection" or "equal rights" under the law. So **equality** refers to the sphere of our lives in which laws and rights are active. This is our political life. In health care, this legal realm of life, especially over the past 150 years, has essentially become an instrument for the economic realm of life to become predominant in society. Through laws today, many people are denied equal access to quality health care. Laws now deny seniors coverage for non-drug therapies that work. Laws also restrict employees from seeking what they feel are appropriate therapies when these are not covered by their insurance plan. These laws prop up excessive, insensitive corporate health care, and often deny access to people with low incomes.

Then we have **liberty.** In the realm of culture, which includes religion, the arts, education, and health care, the key word is liberty, or freedom. Throughout this book are references to how the freedom to choose one's own doctor has been restricted. What then is meant by freedom in the context of health care?

In the United States today, we have put freedom on a pedestal and put responsibility in the gutter. Freedom has come to be equated with license. We think we are free because we can go to a movie or another city anytime we want, or we can eat anything we want and have the burger made the way we want. But these are material freedoms. Though material freedom is not to be taken for granted, as it is restricted in many countries, the way we practice it is freedom taken to its extreme because it lacks boundaries. These boundaries are what we would call responsibility. We want the freedom to eat whatever we want, to do whatever we want, and then have someone else pay for the consequences. This is freedom without responsibility. What we have today is a false and misleading sense of freedom, and entrenched self-centeredness.

A system of healthy medicine is characterized both by freedom of choice in health care practitioner and by all parties involved taking responsibility for the consequences of living in unhealthy ways. For the individual, this means accepting the responsibility for taking care of him or herself. For health care practitioners and suppliers, this responsibility means having transparent finances and making service and support of healing, rather than shareholder profit, their principle reason for existence in the health care field.

The Great Law of Peace in the Iroquois Confederation uses the phrase "autonomous responsibility." This meant that each person judged only him or herself, viewed the others as masters of themselves and their own actions, and let others conduct themselves as they wish. This is what we need again in health care and in the United States in general.

This quality of freedom or liberty is most fully expressed in the cultural realm of life. There is freedom of speech, freedom of religion, freedom of expression. And there is freedom to choose one's own doctor. It is in the cultural sphere of our lives, as opposed to the political or economic arenas, that we most deeply connect with our inner spiritual and human creative needs. When we sit quietly and alone in prayer or meditation, or reading a book, in eating our food, or in taking our medicines, we live in this realm of life.

The true home of health care is in this cultural sphere of our lives, not in the political and economic arenas. It is important that we see this. When we are truly free, we choose the health practitioner with whom we wish to work, which is really no different from choosing a priest for confession, or a teacher or a book through which to learn and grow. All three of these examples are sacred to our most deeply human qualities. It is the work of healing that we undertake when we exercise the right to choose our own practitioner.

But this right must be exercised. Too often today we think healing means making symptoms go away, or eliminating organs surgically. This is not healing, but rather is fixing. If we demand to be fixed, then we will continue to get what we deserve: a sickness care system that will drive us into bankruptcy and in which we feel passively helpless. As earlier generations of great Americans have said, liberty must be fought for. Not on the streets or in overt battles with opposing forces as in the past, but in our own individual lives and local communities. And it is Lady Liberty, who sits in the harbor of our greatest financial center, who is the national symbol for this quality of Freedom. We must bring this Liberty/Freedom into our financial and economic lives, including health care.

A further ideal of the American spirit can be found in the song "America the Beautiful": "And crown thy good with brotherhood from sea to shining sea." **Fraternity,** or brotherhood, is the part of the trinity of Liberty/Equality/Fraternity that is often forgotten. We have become a land of individuals seeking our own profit and protection. The common good is rarely thought of today. And the pursuit of happiness is more often than not a selfish, me-first phenomenon that damages local culture and economy.

A key part of a new and successful health care system, based on the sound principles of healthy medicine, is to support the growth of fraternity in the form of local communities and local economy. Without what author Christopher Budd calls an "enlarged egoism" that is inclusive of others, in which we recognize that our own happiness cannot be gained at the expense of others, we will continue to live in fear of scarcity, poverty, and illness, and lose sight of the abundance that is present all around us. This abundance that we equate with happiness is present when we are guided by the spirit of service and inclusiveness, or what is known as a win-win situation.

To be clear, although health care economics is an important focus of this book, a medical model based in comprehensive medicine recognizes health care as a spiritual cultural endeavor. Through the work of healing, we raise the human spirit and give birth to dormant creativity in every person. This has to be our goal in health care. For this to work effectively, we must establish clear and healthy boundaries between this cultural realm (the true realm of health care), the political realm of laws, and the economic realm of products and services. Healthy Medicine Associations, guided by comprehensive medicine practices and environmental sustainability, are an effort to begin this process.

If we can again establish these healthy boundaries, then, instead of rampant and destructive free-market forces, we can strive to create the conditions whereby life, liberty, and the pursuit of happiness are within reach of all Americans.

BIBLIOGRAPHY

Abramson, John, *Overdo$ed America: The Broken Promise of American Medicine,* New York: HarperCollins, 2004.

Berry, Wendell, *In The Presence of Fear: Three Essays for a Changed World.* Great Barrington, MA: The Orion Society, 2001.

Budd, Christopher Houghton, *Rare Albion: The Further Adventures of the Wizard from Oz: A Monetary Allegory.* London: New Economy Publications, 2005.

Critser, Greg, *Generation Rx: How Prescription Drugs Are Altering American Lives, Minds, and Bodies.* New York: Houghton Mifflin, 2005.

Glover, Paul, *Health Democracy: Liberating Americans from Medical Insurance,* healthdemocracy.org, 2006.

Hadler, Norton M.D. *The Last Well Person: How to Stay Well Despite the Health Care System.* Canada: McGill Queen's University Press, 2004.

Himmelstein, David, M.D., Woolhandler, Steffie, M.D., M.D.H., with Hellander, Ida, M.D., *Bleeding the Patient: The Consequences of Corporate Healthcare.* Monroe, ME: Common Courage Press, 2003.

Twist, Lynn, *The Soul of Money: Transforming Your Relationship with Money and Life.* New York: Norton, 2003.

Wheatley, Margaret, *Finding Our Way: Leadership for an Uncertain Time.* San Francisco: Berrett-Koehler Publishers, 2005.

Zieve, Robert, M.D., *Healthy Medicine: A Guide to the Emergence of Sensible, Comprehensive Care,* Great Barrington, MA: Bell Pond Books, 2005.

THE EMERSON CENTER
FOR HEALTHY MEDICINE

THE EMERSON CENTER for Healthy Medicine, Inc. is a nonprofit collaboration of health care practitioners, economists, community educators, legal professionals, business people, and artists. Our purpose is to develop creative ideas about how to change our health care system and to offer educational support to individuals and groups who seek to improve health care by making it more effective and affordable.

Our mission is to collaborate with others in supporting the new impulse that is emerging today in health care. The goal is to establish a system of healthy medicine that supports all people in real healing and thereby enhances business productivity and community well-being.

For public forums, business groups, and health care institutions striving to make the necessary transition to healthy medicine, we provide:

- Lectures
- Workshops
- Consulting services
- Educational material

To be effective, these changes must be made simultaneously and synchronistically, through well-thought-out plans that at their core are heart-centered and guided by intelligent thinking and the spirit of cooperation. In this way, we create truly therapeutic environments and an economy of healing.

The center is named for the man who has been called America's teacher: Ralph Waldo Emerson. Emerson's writings embody the true spirit of America: self-reliance, individual responsibility, authenticity, and a reverence for nature. These ideals guide us even today and need to form the foundation of our efforts to change health care.

The center's educational and consulting services for transforming a sickness care industry into a healing care collaboration are inspired by the principles Emerson set forth more than 150 years ago. In the past one hundred years, these principles have been forgotten, discarded, and undermined by developments in society as a whole and in the field of health care in particular. It is time to reinvoke the principles of Emerson, Thoreau, and others of their time.

Emerson once said, "The Americans have little faith. They rely on the power of the dollar." The purpose of the Emerson Center is to help restore faith in our health care system by bringing it into alignment again with the Spirit of America. This Spirit has been darkened by fear. The center provides guiding principles to rediscover faith and hope in life and health.

Emerson Center for Healthy Medicine, Inc.
P.O. Box 11235
Prescott, AZ 86304
Tel: (928) 778-7047
Fax: (928) 778-3515
Email: info@healthymedicine.org
Website: www.healthymedicine.org

About the Author

ROBERT J. ZIEVE, M.D., is the director of Pine Tree Clinic for Comprehensive Medicine in Prescott, Arizona, and is a participating physician in the Integrative Medical Healing Center in Scottsdale. His practice includes homeopathy, European biological medicine, anthroposophical medicine, and nutrition.

A graduate of the Ohio State University College of Medicine, Dr. Zieve has served as a board-certified specialist in emergency medicine, an emergency department director, and medical director of Paracelsus Foxhollow Clinic, a comprehensive biological medicine clinic in Louisville, Kentucky. He is a past-president of the Arizona Homeopathic and Integrative Medical Association.

Dr. Zieve is also an author and lecturer. He has lectured on the subject of alternative medicine to groups in both clinical orthodox medicine and holistic medicine for more than twenty years, both locally and nationally. He is the author of *Healthy Medicine: A Guide to the Emergence of Sensible Comprehensive Care,* among other books. Dr. Zieve is currently president of the non-profit organization, The Emerson Center for Healthy Medicine, Inc. (www.healthymedicine.org)

Printed in the United States
59491LVS00002B/172-246

9 780880 105729